Practical social work

**Published in conjunction with
the British Association of Social Workers**

Founding editor: Jo Campling

Social Work is a multi-skilled profession, centred on people. Social workers need skills in problem-solving, communication, critical reflection and working with others to be effective in practice.

The British Association of Social Workers (www.basw.co.uk) has always been conscious of its role in setting guidelines for practice and in seeking to raise professional standards. The concept of the Practical Social Work series was developed to fulfil a genuine professional need for a carefully planned, coherent, series of texts that would contribute to practitioners' skills, development and professionalism.

Newly relaunched to meet the ever-changing needs of the social work profession, the series has been reviewed and revised with the help of the BASW Editorial Advisory Board:

Peter Beresford
Jim Campbell
Monica Dowling
Brian Littlechild
Mark Lymbery
Fraser Mitchell
Steve Moore

Under their guidance each book marries practice issues with theory and research in a compact and applied format: perfect for students, practitioners and educators.

A comprehensive list of titles available in the series can be found online at: www.palgrave.com/socialwork/basw

Series standing order **ISBN 0–333–80313–2**

You can receive future titles in this series as they are published by placing a standing order. Please contact your bookseller or, in the case of difficulty, contact us at the address below with your name and address, the title of the series and the ISBN quoted above.

Customer Services Department, Macmillan Distribution Ltd, Houndmills, Basingstoke, Hampshire RG21 6XS, England

Practical Social Work Series

Founding Editor: Jo Campling

New and best-selling titles

ANTI-DISCRIMINATORY PRACTICE

Equality, Diversity and Social Justice

Sixth Edition

NEIL THOMPSON

 macmillan education   palgrave

First edition 1992
Second edition 1997
Third edition 2001
Fourth edition 2006
Fifth edition 2012
Sixth edition 2016

Published by
PALGRAVE.

Palgrave in the UK is an imprint of Macmillan Publishers Limited, registered in England, company number 785998, of 4 Crinan Street, London, N1 9XW.

Palgrave® and Macmillan® are registered trademarks in the United States, the United Kingdom, Europe and other countries.

ISBN 978–1–137–58665–0 paperback

This book is printed on paper suitable for recycling and made from fully managed and sustained forest sources. Logging, pulping and manufacturing processes are expected to conform to the environmental regulations of the country of origin.

A catalogue record for this book is available from the British Library.

A catalog record for this book is available from the Library of Congress.

Printed by CPI Group (UK) Ltd, Croydon CR0 4YY

For Susan and Anna

BRIEF CONTENTS

CONTENTS

LIST OF FIGURES

PREFACE

In the Preface to the fourth edition of this book, I wrote: 'When a book reaches its fourth edition, it is a sure sign that it has achieved a significant measure of success'. The fact that this is now the sixth edition clearly reinforces that message.

This is partly, no doubt, due to the importance of social justice and a commitment to tackling discrimination and oppression as basic social work values and partly – if the feedback I have received is to be believed – because the book presents a clear and helpful picture of the complexities of developing anti-discriminatory practice and provides a foundation of understanding that casts important light on how we can rise to the challenges involved.

It is now almost twenty-five years since I started writing the first edition of this book. Times have changed a great deal during that period and we have made some significant advances in tackling discrimination and oppression. However, the challenges we face remain enormous and represent a long-term project. At the time of writing the first edition I was a team manager in a social services department and in daily contact with many of the issues covered in this book. For over eighteen years my role as a trainer and consultant brought me into almost daily contact with practitioners, managers, students and educators who are wrestling with the challenges of ensuring that social work interventions are positive and empowering, rather than disempowering and demeaning. I am therefore very aware that there is a need for this book and that it has an important part to play.

Despite the fact that some writers have misrepresented my work (see Chapter 9), such distortions have not prevented this text in its various incarnations from helping generation after generation of social workers to appreciate the importance of tackling discrimination and oppression and providing a foundation of basic understanding on which to build over time. This new edition has been developed to build on that success and to keep these vitally important issues firmly on the agenda.

The aim is of the book remains to locate anti-discriminatory practice in the context of equality, diversity and social justice. A key point I want to get across is that, while 'anti-discriminatory practice' is a long-established term in the social work vocabulary (some might even see it as old-fashioned now), the ideas on which it is based are as relevant and pressing now as they were decades ago. The introduction of new terminology and new ideas should be seen as part of the development of anti-discriminatory practice as a vibrant field and not as a replacement for it.

This book was written specifically with a social work readership in mind. However, I have become aware that it is also widely used by others within the human services or helping professions (for example, nurses, advice workers, probation officers and youth and community workers). It is to be hoped that readers in this latter category will not find the constant references to social work too discouraging. Tutors and others involved in supporting learning may find it helpful to encourage readers, whenever they encounter the term 'social work' to stop and think about how the point being made applies to their own professional discipline. In many cases it may be very similar, but this will not always be the case. Making these comparisons between social work and their own discipline can be an important part of learning.

Whether the book is used in its originally intended field of social work or in what has become its wider constituency of the people professions more broadly defined, it remains an *introductory* text. This book has a number of important messages to put across, but it remains the case, of course, that a short introductory book like this cannot realistically incorporate our knowledge base in anything approaching a comprehensive or exhaustive way. The more in-depth book, *Promoting Equality* (Thompson, 2011a) takes the issues further, but even that cannot address all the issues involved in this complex area of theory and practice. References at various points in this book to *Promoting Equality* relate to that book. It is perhaps helpful to see *Anti-Discriminatory Practice* as a first-level, introductory text, while *Promoting Equality* is a follow-on text, for readers looking to explore more deeply and widely. Indeed, the issues covered in this book are so important that it is essential to go beyond the basics and to read more widely and tackle more in-depth texts on specific aspects or forms of discrimination.

In the Preface to the third edition of this book, I made the following comment:

> Throughout the process of writing this book there has been no doubt in my mind that its role is as an *introductory* text, a gateway to the broader and more advanced literature. It is certainly not intended as an 'all you need to know on the subject' type of book. I have therefore found it quite

sad, especially as an external examiner at various universities, to note so many students using the book as if it were the only one available on the subject! I am, of course, pleased that the book has become established as a key text, but this does not alter the fact that it is a key *introductory* text and should therefore not be used as a substitute for reading more widely or for engaging with the more advanced texts available. ... If you find this book helpful, then that's great, but please use any benefits you have gained from it as a launch pad for further learning, and not as a source of complacency that stands in the way of further development.

I still wish to reinforce that message as I continue to see the potential problem of the book's strengths becoming a weakness by discouraging further reading and learning. I hope that tutors, trainers and practice learning staff will play their part by emphasizing this point.

Each of the main chapters ends with a short guide to further reading relating to the subject matter of that particular chapter. There is also a guide to further learning to be found online as part of the Palgrave Macmillan website, *The Effective Social Worker* (www.palgrave.com/the-effective-social-worker). This site is well worth consulting.

To prevent any unnecessary confusion, I feel it is important to clarify two issues relating to the use of terminology. First, at one time it became the practice of some people to distinguish between anti-discriminatory and anti-oppressive practice. For such commentators, the former was reserved for a narrow, legalistic perspective that did not take on board wider sociopolitical concerns. It is therefore important to clarify, right from the start, that this is not a distinction I shall be drawing here. As the arguments presented in this book should make very clear, I adopt a holistic perspective on anti-discriminatory practice – that is, I see it as a broad undertaking that needs to incorporate sociological, political and economic concerns above and beyond narrow legal requirements. In my view, discrimination is the process (or set of processes) that leads to oppression. To challenge oppression, it is therefore necessary to challenge discrimination. Anti-discriminatory and anti-oppressive practice are therefore presented here as more or less synonymous terms, on the grounds that a legalistic perspective is too narrow to challenge discrimination and the ensuing oppression, and does not therefore merit the title of 'anti-discriminatory'. I shall revisit this point in Chapter 1.

Second, the term 'client' is one that I use throughout this book and indeed in many of my writings. It is important to recognize that this is a contested term. Many people have abandoned it in favour of 'service user'. However, many people object to this latter term, especially when it is shortened to 'user'. In my view, client is a term of respect and is consistent with the notion of professionalism (see Thompson, 2009a, for a fuller discussion of this). In addition, in view of the growing critique of 'consumerist' approaches to social work that focus narrowly on service provision (at the expense of social work's wider problem-solving and empowerment roles), we need to be aware that the term 'service user' reinforces a consumerist perspective. It is for this reason that the term 'citizen' is now being increasingly used, especially in Wales.

Finally, I am hopeful that you will find this revised and updated edition both interesting and useful and that it will serve as an important foundation for developing your knowledge and understanding further.

Neil Thompson

ACKNOWLEDGEMENTS

In developing this new edition I have once again had the support and assistance of a good many people. My thanks go yet again to those who provided helpful comments in the development of the original edition – their contributions continue to be of value.

It has become something of a habit for me to express my gratitude to Dr Susan Thompson for her unwavering support – moral, practical and intellectual. That continues to be the case for this edition. I would be lost without her.

Other friends who have helped in the development of my thinking and whose influence can be seen here are Denise Bevan of the Hospice of the Good Shepherd, Chester, Dr John Bates, formerly of Liverpool Hope University, Bernard Moss, Emeritus Professor, Staffordshire University and Colin Richardson, Fellow of Keele University.

Peter Hooper at the publishers has proven to be very helpful and supportive whenever called upon. I would also like to say thank you to the very many participants on courses I have run over the years who have shared their experiences and views with me and who have reaffirmed my commitment to developing forms of education and training geared towards tackling discrimination and oppression which are not in themselves oppressive.

This edition follows the pattern of the first five in that it is dedicated to Susan and Anna, the two most important people in my life.

THE AUTHOR

Neil Thompson is an independent writer and online tutor. He has held full or honorary professorships at four UK universities and has over 38 years' experience in the people professions as a practitioner, manager, educator and consultant. He has 35 books to his name. These include:

Power and Empowerment (Russell House Publishing, 2007)
The Critically Reflective Practitioner (with Sue Thompson, Palgrave Macmillan, 2008)
Promoting Equality: Working with Diversity and Difference (Palgrave Macmillan, 3rd edn, 2011)
Effective Communication (Palgrave Macmillan, 2nd edn, 2011)
The People Solutions Sourcebook (Palgrave Macmillan, 2nd edn, 2012)
People Management (Palgrave Macmillan, 2013)
People Skills (Palgrave Macmillan, 4th edn, 2015)
The Authentic Leader (Palgrave Macmillan, 2016)

He is also involved in writing a growing number of e-books, including *A Career in Social Work*; *How to Do Social Work*; and *Effective Writing*.

Another important part of Neil's work is the development of a range of other learning resources, including training manuals, DVDs, e-learning courses, e-mentoring (www.avenuelearningcentre.co.uk) and the innovative online learning community, the Avenue Professional Development Programme, which is a form of online tutorial group geared towards promoting continuous professional development, based on supported self-directed learning principles (www.apdp.org.uk).

He has qualifications in: social work; management (MBA); training and development; mediation and dispute resolution; as well as a first-class honours degree in social sciences, a doctorate (PhD) and a higher doctorate (DLitt). His PhD and DLitt focused on existentialism. Neil is a Fellow of the Chartered Institute of Personnel and Development and the Royal Society of Arts, elected to the latter on the basis of his contribution to workplace learning. He is also a Fellow of the Higher Education Academy and a Life Fellow of the Institute of Welsh Affairs. He was the founding editor of the *British Journal of Occupational Learning* and was also previously the editor of the US-based international journal, *Illness, Crisis & Loss*. He currently edits the free e-zines, **THE** *humansolutions* **BULLETIN** and *Learning IMPACT* (www.neilthompson.info/connect). His personal website and blog are at www.neilthompson.info.

INTRODUCTION

During the late 1980s social work education became increasingly aware of the impact of oppression and discrimination on clients and communities. There was a growing awareness and recognition of the relative neglect of such issues in traditional approaches to social work. This emphasis on combating discrimination is part of the process of establishing an awareness of discrimination and a commitment to challenging it as fundamental building blocks of qualifying training and subsequent practice. They were therefore seen as an essential part of the curriculum and the evaluation process and continue to be regarded as such, as is shown by their inclusion in the curriculum for the current qualifying programmes in social work.

This major development in education and training has also been reflected more broadly, to a certain extent at least, in social work policy, theory and practice (although it would be naïve not to acknowledge that much progress remains to be made in these respects). Anti-discriminatory practice has therefore been featuring as a regular and high priority item on the social work agenda for some time now, although there sadly continues to be a great deal of misunderstanding and oversimplification of the issues.

But it is not only students as new entrants to the profession who need a grounding in the theory and practice of anti-discriminatory social work. There remain very many practitioners, managers and trainers who can benefit from developing a fuller understanding of the complexities involved and begin to appreciate that we need to wrestle constantly with these issues, rather than find some sort of easy answer or ultimate resolution.

The primary aim of this book is to provide just such a grounding – for qualified staff, for those seeking qualification, for practice teachers, trainers and managers and for others with a general interest in contemporary social work, equality and diversity or related issues. The text seeks to clarify and to answer, in part at least, a number of important questions:

- What are the factors underlying discrimination and oppression, especially as they relate to social work theory and practice?

- What are the common concepts and issues across the various forms of discrimination – sexism, racism, ageism and so on? What are the key differences?

- Why is the development of anti-discriminatory practice so important?

- What are the necessary steps towards constructing a social work practice based on principles of anti-discrimination and the promotion of equality?

The idea of anti-discriminatory practice has now become very well established in social work and has become part of mainstream thinking to a large extent. This does not mean that there is much more for us to learn, much more for us to do. Dropping our guard and slipping backwards to the days when discrimination was not taken seriously is a pitfall we must clearly avoid. This is particularly important in view of the increasing inequality brought about by wider social, political and economic factors in the current climate (Dorling, 2014; Hills, 2015; Jones, 2015; Stiglitz, 2013). Despite the progress made in developing our awareness of discrimination and oppression and developing anti-discriminatory approaches to theory, policy, practice and education, there is no room for complacency. We continue to face major challenges when it comes to promoting equality and enabling social work to make a contribution to a more humane and equitable society.

Structure and outline

In the first chapter, I discuss the key underlying concepts of equality, diversity and social justice. I show that these are not only concepts, in an intellectual sense, but also values in a practice sense – that is, principles that can and should guide our actions. I argue that we cannot really understand discrimination and oppression without first having a good understanding of these three key issues. Another major feature of this chapter is the emphasis I place on the argument that unfair discrimination is something that needs to be tackled in all its forms and not only the more well-established ones or more fully documented ones. Anti-discriminatory practice is a matter of a principled commitment to equality, diversity and social justice, rather than simply following political, intellectual or other fashions.

Chapter 2 examines a range of other theoretical concepts that can be seen to underpin anti-discriminatory practice. The major themes are explained and links with social work practice are drawn in order to begin to build a bridge between theory and practice. Indeed, the need for a clear practice focus, illuminated by theory, will be a primary concern throughout the book (Thompson, 2000a; 2010). This chapter will also tackle the thorny issue of language. The topic will be approached from two angles: first, to understand the role played by language in constructing and reinforcing discrimination; and, second, to clarify the terminology used in this text – that is, to define the key terms and concepts.

This chapter sets the scene for the following analysis of the various forms of oppression and processes of discrimination. This is achieved by explaining the common theory base which acts as a framework for understanding the complex issues discussed in ensuing chapters. Chapter 3 is the first of six chapters to explore a specific area of discrimination, in this case gender. The theory of patriarchy is explained and the steps towards an anti-sexist practice are sketched out. Chapters 4 to 8 follow a similar structure and pattern. Chapter 4 addresses issues of race/ethnicity and racism. Imperialist ideology and notions of cultural superiority are explored and rejected as a first step towards building a social work practice based on principles of anti-racism. In Chapter 5 the less publicized and less well-established concept of ageism is the object of our attention. The issues of discrimination on the grounds of age are considered and a framework for developing anti-ageist practice is presented. Chapter 6 adopts a similar approach in exploring the marginalization of disabled people. Discriminatory attitudes, policies, structures and practices are identified and the oppression inherent in catering only for the able-bodied majority is recognized as a target for change.

In Chapter 7 attention is paid to discrimination on the grounds of sexual identity (heterosexism). Here the focus is on how social work needs to take account of how sexuality can be a basis for unfair treatment of individuals and groups. Chapter 8 is concerned with religious discrimination. It explores how matters of faith, sect and political outlook intertwine to produce a complex situation characterized by discrimination. The chapter argues that social workers need to be aware of these issues if they are to avoid making the situation worse.

Chapter 9 is the concluding chapter. It summarizes seven main themes and examines possible ways forward, divided into seven positive steps to be taken and seven pitfalls to avoid. The focus here is on the need to develop critically reflective practice (Thompson and Thompson, 2008) – that is, forms of practice that incorporate a critical evaluation of our own actions. This is necessary to ensure that social work is part of the solution, rather than part of the problem.

Important note

Each of the main chapters has a Further resources section and there is also a References section at the end of the book (see also www.palgrave.com/the-effective-social-worker). Please note that the inclusion of particular publications or websites in these sections means that I feel they are worth consulting. However, this does not mean that I necessarily agree with and endorse everything the authors concerned put forward in their writings or on their websites.

CHAPTER 1

EQUALITY, DIVERSITY AND SOCIAL JUSTICE

CHAPTER OVERVIEW

In this chapter you will:

- Learn more about the key concept of discrimination and why it is so important in social work and related professional disciplines
- Start to understand how anti-discriminatory practice is underpinned by a commitment to equality, diversity and social justice
- Appreciate the importance of moving away from medicalized approaches to personal and social problems which oversimplify complex issues

Introduction

People are different, in the sense that the population in general and social work's clientele in particular are characterized by immense diversity. Where there is difference, there is the potential for unfair discrimination, in so far as it creates the potential for particular individuals or groups to be identified as 'different' and therefore treated less favourably (I will return to this point below). Anti-discriminatory practice is, or should be, more than simply tackling those well-publicized areas of discrimination and oppression that attract considerable attention – it should encompass all forms of discrimination that can be seen to lead to disadvantage, disempowerment and oppression. That is, we need to adopt a *holistic* approach to discrimination and related matters, rather than a narrow or partial one.

The managing diversity approach (as represented in the work of Kandola and Fullerton, 1998) is one of the models we will explore in more detail below. However, for now, we can note that it can be criticized for being too individualistic and paying inadequate attention to cultural and structural levels of discrimination and is therefore not sufficiently holistic. However, one of its strong points is that it acknowledges:

- the significance of diversity (that is, variety across individuals and groups of people) and the need to affirm and value it;
- that differences between people can and should be seen as assets to be appreciated, rather than problems to be solved; and
- that difference can so easily lead to unfair discrimination.

Diversity is therefore an important concept that we need to take seriously but, as we shall see, we need to make sure that it is not oversimplified or seen as an easy answer (Malik, 2008). As von Mende and Houlihan (2007) comment:

> The persistence of discrimination, inequalities and power differences suggests that the rhetoric of diversity can be criticized as sanitizing difference, and simply masking or attenuating underlying conflicts (Netmetz and Christensen, 1996).
>
> (von Mende and Houlihan, 2007, p. 217)

Race, ethnicity, gender, class, sexual identity, age, language, disability, religion and so on are just some of the dimensions of diversity and therefore just some of the ways in which difference can so easily be translated into discrimination and oppression as a result of the various power-related processes to be discussed in later chapters. However, these are not only dimensions of diversity in a sociological sense, they are also dimensions of experience in a psychological sense. That is, each sociologically defined area of discrimination can be analysed and explored as a discrete aspect of the social world. However, to each individual person, these are not discrete areas, they are very real intertwined dimensions of experience, part and parcel of our lived experience (what is often referred to by the French technical term, 'le vécu') and have to be understood as such. That is, the reality for each person is having to deal with a complex set of interactions across perhaps several of these different areas, rather than simply encountering discrete, unconnected areas to be considered in isolation.

This means, in effect, that we must consider each situation in its own right, rather than apply general principles in an oversimplified and dogmatic way. We must not make assumptions about 'men' or 'black people' or 'disabled people' or 'Welsh speakers', but rather consider each unique individual in the context of what we know of the influences and implications of these broad categories and their sociological significance – to link the social level of context to the personal level of unique individual experience (Thompson, 2012), rather than fall into one of the two disastrous, but none the less common traps of either (i) treating unique individuals as if they were simply non-specific examples of social categories; or (ii) failing to recognize that individuals are unique partly because of the diversity of the social context that plays a part in shaping all of our experiences.

It should be clear, then, that discrimination is not a simple matter and that it would therefore be both inappropriate and dangerous to adopt an oversimplified approach to the challenges of developing anti-discriminatory practice. We therefore need to develop quite a sophisticated level of understanding of the complexities involved, rather than look for simple solutions that can be both woefully inadequate (in terms of not doing justice to the intricacies of what we are dealing with) and potentially disastrous (in terms of making the situation worse). It is for this reason that the first two chapters of the book concentrate on developing a platform for building up a theoretical understanding of discrimination and related concepts so that we are able to begin to face the demands of anti-discriminatory practice in an informed way.

In the first of these two scene-setting chapters we explore some key concepts before, in Chapter 2, examining a particular theoretical framework that can pull together our understanding of discrimination. Understandably, we begin our discussion of the key concepts with discrimination itself. We then move on to look at the three very important concepts that form the subtitle of the book, namely equality, diversity and social justice. This leads into a consideration of oppression, the negative and unwelcome results of discrimination (Mullaly, 2002). Finally, we examine the need to avoid 'medicalization', a process of pathologizing individuals that has highly discriminatory – and thus oppressive – consequences.

Voice of experience 1.1
_____

I used to work in a team that thought that all the talk about discrimination was a load of nonsense. It was hard work trying to get them to see that so many of the situations they were dealing with involved one or more forms of discrimination. We had to discuss it at several team meetings before people could see just how important it was. *Viv, manager of a hospital social work team*

What is discrimination?

The literal meaning of the term 'to discriminate' is to identify a difference. As such it is not necessarily a negative term. For example, being able to discriminate between safe food and harmful poison is clearly a good thing. However, when the term is used in a legal, moral or political sense (as in this book), it is generally used to refer to *unfair* discrimination. That is, it refers to the process (or set of processes) through which (i) a difference is identified; and (ii) that difference is used as the basis of unfair treatment. To use the technical term, a person or group 'suffers a detriment' (that is, experiences a disadvantage) because they are identified as 'different' (in terms of gender, race/ethnicity, sexual identity and so on) in ways that are deemed to be socially and/or politically significant.

Instead of differences between people being seen as positive (as per the diversity approach mentioned above and to be discussed more fully below), they become the basis of unfair discrimination, a basis for disadvantaging certain groups of people. This discrimination then becomes a source of oppression. It is through the process of identifying some people as 'different' that they receive inhuman or degrading treatment (a key part of the definition of oppression we will explore more fully in Chapter 2) and are thus oppressed.

While this is a satisfactory basic definition of discrimination, what it does not do is indicate the important role of power that is involved. Anyone can discriminate against anyone else. However, where the impact will be of major proportions is in those cases where relatively powerful groups will be in a position to discriminate systematically (whether directly or indirectly) against those in relatively powerless groups (Dalrymple and Burke, 2006). Such power can arise because of personal circumstances or characteristics, cultural norms or structural position (in Chapter 2 we will look at these dimensions of power in more detail). This is where established patterns of discrimination have become ingrained in social practices – racism, sexism, ageism and so on, and are not simply examples of individual preference or prejudice.

Discrimination is therefore a sociological and political phenomenon as well as a psychological one, hence the need for a holistic approach, as mentioned earlier.

Practice focus 1.1

Lynne was a psychology graduate who had recently begun her social work training on a postgraduate course. From the sociology component of the course, she began to appreciate how narrow her perspective had previously been. She began to realize that, although her psychological perspective was very important and valuable, she also needed to understand the wider sociological issues that were

▶

> so relevant to the life experiences of social work clients, relationships between social workers and clients and so on. She had begun to develop the 'sociological imagination'.

Note that, in referring to power, I was very careful to use the term 'relatively'. This is because, as we shall see below, there has been a tendency to oversimplify issues of power and reduce them to a simple dichotomy of two groups in society: the powerful and the powerless. Power is a much more complex phenomenon than this, and so it is important, at this early stage in our discussions, not to fall into the trap of presenting it too simply (see Thompson, 2007, for a fuller explanation of the significance of power and the complexities associated with it).

A key point to note is that the model of anti-discriminatory practice presented here is not a narrow one that ignores important wider sociopolitical concerns. In the early days of putting discrimination and oppression on the social work agenda some people conceptualized anti-discriminatory practice in narrow, legalistic terms – a very different approach from the one that I am adopting, and advocating, here.

Good practice is anti-discriminatory practice

Social workers can be seen as mediators between their clients and the wider state apparatus and social order. This position of 'mediator' is a crucial one, as it means that social workers are in a pivotal position in terms of the relationship between the state and its citizens (Ferguson and Woodward, 2009).

The relationship is a double-edged one, consisting of elements of care and control. It is also double-edged in the sense that it can lead to either potential empowerment or potential oppression – social work interventions can help or hinder, empower or oppress. Which aspect is to the fore, which element or tendency is reinforced depends largely on the actions of the social workers concerned. As long ago as 1975, in the era of radical social work, Peter Leonard captured this point in relation to class and capitalism, although much the same can be said of gender and patriarchy, race and imperialism and so on:

> In capitalist society, social work operates as part of a social-welfare system which is located at the centre of the contradictions arising from

the dehumanizing consequences of capitalist economic production. Social workers, although situated in a largely oppressive organizational and professional context, have the potential for recognizing these contradictions and, through working at the point of interaction between people and their social environment, of helping to increase the control by people over economic and political structures.

(Leonard, 1975, p. 55)

What this entails, in effect, is that there can be no safe middle ground, no simple compromise. This differs significantly from the traditional approach to such matters. Social work is not, as Halmos (1965) would have it, a matter of the personal detached from the political (Pearson, 1975).

As I argued many years ago:

There is no middle ground; intervention either adds to oppression (or at least condones it) or goes some small way towards easing or breaking such oppression. In this respect, the political slogan, 'If you're not part of the solution, you must be part of the problem' is particularly accurate. An awareness of the sociopolitical context is necessary in order to prevent becoming (or remaining) part of the problem.

(Thompson, 1992, pp. 169–70)

In short, a social work practice that does not take account of oppression, and the discrimination that gives rise to it, cannot be seen as good practice, no matter how high its standards may be in other respects. For example, a social work intervention with a disabled person that fails to recognize the marginalized position of disabled people in society runs the risk of doing the client more of a disservice than a service (see Chapter 6).

Key point 1.1

When it comes to discrimination and oppression, there is no neutral middle ground. If we are not challenging the unfair ways people are treated, then at best we are implicitly condoning them and may actually be reinforcing them.

This principle – that good practice must be anti-discriminatory practice – should become more clearly and firmly established in the chapters that follow.

A sophisticated understanding of discrimination is called for

One unfortunate development that accompanied the growing awareness of, and commitment to, anti-discriminatory practice, was a strong tendency towards oversimplification or 'reductionism' – reducing a complex, multi-level phenomenon to a simple, single-level issue language use and discrimination became reduced to 'political correctness' – a reliance on a list of taboo or 'non-PC' words (see Thompson, 2011b). This was also accompanied in many quarters by a very crude approach to education and training in relation to discrimination and oppression, a point to which we shall return in Chapter 2. This crude reductionism, while a significant problem in its own right, also led to another major concern – the development of a culture of fear and blame in which defensiveness became a very common response. It is understandable that if students and in-service course participants were being told in effect that they were 'oppressive', they were likely to perceive this as an attack and thus respond in a defensive manner. Key features of this defensiveness have been:

- A tokenistic 'lip-service' approach caused by people's understandable reluctance to engage firmly and closely with what they perceived as such dangerous, threatening issues.

- A tendency to avoid the subject where possible – a 'Let's not go there' mentality.

- A tense and anxious approach which in itself could lead to oversimplification (when we feel tense, anxious and threatened, we are not likely to be eager to engage with very complex and intricate concepts and issues).

- In some cases, a long-standing lack of confidence in dealing with these issues as a result of the painful experiences of being exposed to some very crude and ill-thought-through approaches to teaching and learning (Thompson, 2009b).

In running courses on the subject of anti-discriminatory practice I have come across large numbers of people who have given me very worrying examples of earlier experiences that were extremely unhelpful in contributing to their understanding of the complexities or in equipping them to deal with such issues effectively in practice. This is a sad legacy of a rapid change from an education and training system which largely neglected discrimination and oppression to one in which such concerns very quickly became central. It is to be hoped that we have managed to learn the lessons from that period and are now adopting much more sophisticated approaches not only to anti-discriminatory practice itself, but also to how such matters are addressed through education and training.

It is therefore to be hoped that we can develop a sophisticated level of understanding of discrimination and related matters that goes beyond the dogmatic and oversimplified levels of understanding that have stood in the way of progress at various times in the past (and still manifest themselves occasionally to this day). Malik, for example, is critical of what Penketh (2000) calls 'the excesses of anti-racism':

> The concept of race is irrational. The practice of antiracism has become so. We need to challenge both, in the name of humanism and of reason.
>
> (Malik, 2008, p.288)

I would prefer to challenge such excesses in the name of humanity, rather than humanism, but the argument remains an important one. The point is not that challenging discrimination (whether racism or any other form) is in itself irrational, but rather that we have to guard against overzealous, poorly thought through approaches that run the risk of making the situation worse and giving anti-discriminatory practice a bad name ('political correctness gone mad') (Thompson, 2009b).

Equality

Much of the confusion and oversimplification relating to discrimination over the years can be traced back to a tendency to interpret the term 'equality' too literally. In a mathematical sense, equality means sameness. For example, to say that $2 + 2 = 4$ is to say that 2 plus 2 is the same as (or amounts to) 4. However, we need to remember that, in a social work (and, indeed, a broader social policy) context, we are using the term in a moral or political sense and not a mathematical or literal sense. As Witcher aptly puts it: 'The vision is not for a stagnant pool of sameness. Equality does not have to mean "the same". It can also mean equivalent: different but of equal worth' (2015, p. 11). It is therefore essential to be clear that to promote equality does not mean to promote sameness or to discourage people from being different in any way. Indeed, as we will see later in this chapter, it is quite the opposite of that.

In *Promoting Equality* I make the point that it is more helpful to understand equality to mean equal fairness. What it amounts to is that to recognize that the fact that certain people are 'different from ...' other groups or the mainstream should not be confused with the idea that they are 'less than ...' others. Difference and inferiority (or 'deficit' as some writers put it – see, for example, Valencia, 1997) are not the same thing and we do a considerable disservice to members of minority groups if we fail to recognize this or allow our actions and attitudes to be based on confusing the two terms. As Baker et al. put it: 'all human beings have equal worth and importance, and are therefore equally worthy of concern and respect' (2004, p. 23).

In a sense, equality can be understood to mean an absence of discrimination. If, as we noted above, discrimination involves identifying a difference and then treating people less favourably because of that difference, then clearly this involves a considerable degree of unfairness – people who are being discriminated against are not being treated with equal fairness. We should therefore note that promoting equality and pursuing anti-discriminatory practice are very much the same endeavour.

Equality can be seen to be an important concept at both a broader (macro) level of social policy and the more specific (micro) level of actual practice. In terms of the macro level of policy, the work of Wilkinson and Pickett (2009) is very significant. Based on research spanning 30 years the authors provide a strong argument that the more equal a society is in economic terms (that is, the smaller the gap between the richest and the poorest), the fewer the social problems there will be, the more positive the social relations will be and the higher the levels of well-being will be. One of the key implications of this is that greater equality will benefit not only the poorest in society, but also society as a whole.

In terms of the micro level of practice, discrimination is likely to be an important factor in a high proportion of the situations social workers encounter. Consider the following:

- Children looked after by foster carers or in residential care being discriminated against simply because they are 'in care'.

- Older people being patronized and treated like children because of ageist assumptions.

- People with mental health problems being stigmatized and kept at arm's length, thereby being denied opportunities for full participation in society.

- Disabled people being excluded from certain opportunities because it is assumed that they are incapable.

- Black individuals and families not receiving services because it is assumed that 'they look after their own'.

- A gay teenager not having their sexuality accepted and validated.

- Work with families being based on sexist stereotypes.

This, of course, is not an exhaustive list, but it should be sufficient to establish that discrimination is something that needs to be taken seriously in social work, and indeed the helping professions more broadly. So, at both macro and micro levels, equality is a fundamental concept for social work.

Diversity

One development in recent years that has given us a foundation from which to counter the defensiveness I discussed above is the emergence of the 'diversity approach'. This is a relatively new way of addressing inequality that has become a mainstream approach in many areas, both within and outside social work. It is characterized by two main themes:

1   It adopts a positive approach by emphasizing that diversity (that is, variety and difference) is not only a very real characteristic of contemporary social and organizational life, it is also a *valuable* characteristic. Diversity is seen as an asset, a positive feature of society that enriches our experience – it is something that should be valued, affirmed and even celebrated (Parekh, 2006). The fact that there are differences across ethnic groups, identities, approaches and perspectives should be seen as a good thing, a source of learning, variety, stimulation and interest, rather than a source of unfair discrimination based on 'punishing' some people for being different from the perceived mainstream (for being 'deviant' in some way).

2   It adopts a broad approach by arguing that any form of unfair discrimination is a problem to be tackled (this is a point to which we shall return below), regardless of whether the discrimination in question is illegal or not. In this respect, the diversity approach goes far beyond the traditional equal opportunities approach which tends to limit itself largely to ensuring legal compliance with anti-discrimination legislation (Barry, 2005).

By adopting a positive focus and not limiting itself to legal compliance, the diversity approach has the potential to offer, in part at least, an 'antidote' to the negative and defensive approach which has been allowed to develop in many organizational settings. In this respect, it can be seen as a positive step forward.

However, we should not be too enthusiastic in our embracing of this approach, as it has its down sides too. First, it has the potential to become a return to simplistic approaches to multiculturalism (as discussed in Barry, 2001) which emphasize the positives of cultural diversity, but without acknowledging the realities of how oppressive discrimination can be – that is, it rightly values *diversity*, but without paying adequate attention to the realities of *adversity* for those people subjected to unfair discrimination.

Second, the diversity approach has so far tended to have a very individualistic focus. There is a danger that the gains made in moving away from a psychological approach based on notions of prejudice to a more sophisticated sociological one, based on personal, cultural and structural factors (see Chapter 2) will be lost by an overemphasis on individual factors.

To be fair to the diversity approach, there is nothing inherent within it that makes these problems inevitable – they are dangers rather than necessary flaws. It has to be recognized that the diversity approach is still relatively in its infancy and is in a fairly underdeveloped state. How it develops in the coming years will be very significant.

꒰ Another development in the recent history of anti-discriminatory practice in the United Kingdom is a new wave of anti-discrimination legislation, culminating in the Equality Act 2010. While this is a positive and very welcome step, we have to bear in mind that the role the law can play is always going to be quite limited (consider, for example, the fact that theft is illegal does not prevent it from being widespread as a phenomenon). As we shall see in the chapters that follow, a genuine commitment to anti-discriminatory practice must go far beyond the confines of a narrow, legalistic approach that fails to take account of the wider picture. Moss helps us to understand that a commitment to promoting equality, diversity and social justice is a *values* commitment, rather than a simple matter of applying the law: ꒱

> It is not enough to provide a legal framework: society has to own and celebrate the value base which it seeks to live by. And, as we have seen in our discussions of anti-discriminatory practice, there are fundamental challenges to this value base running through society. It is going to take more than some legal adjustments, however crucial these may be, to reach the situation where everyone in the community is not only valued and

treated with dignity, but where their difference and diversity is celebrated as an enrichment to the community which would otherwise be immeasurably the poorer.

(Moss, 2007, p. 60)

The diversity approach therefore helps us to go beyond approaches that focus narrowly on legal compliance. However, as we shall see in Chapter 2, while this is a step in the right direction, it is not enough on its own.

Social justice

Social justice is another important dimension of anti-discriminatory practice, and so it is important to be clear about what we mean by this key concept.

We can identify two approaches to, or understandings of, social justice: narrow and broad. The narrow conception is concerned with the redistribution of wealth and is associated with a traditional focus on class inequalities and the primacy of economic inequality. Here there is a major emphasis on poverty and the need to eradicate, or at least alleviate it (Lister, 2004). This is parallel with the idea of challenging 'social exclusion' which tends to be discussed in narrow class-based terms relating to income and other economic factors, paying relatively little attention to how other social processes, largely unconnected with class, can also result in exclusion and marginalization (that is, being pushed to the margins of society). Disability discrimination would be a good example of this. The broader approach is concerned with a much wider range of social inequalities: gender, 'race', age, disability, religion, language, sexuality and, indeed, any form of inequality based on social categories (or 'social divisions' to use the technical term) (Barry, 2005).

It is this latter, broader and more holistic sense of social justice that anti-discriminatory practice is concerned with (Ferguson, 2008).

Thompson and Thompson capture the importance of social justice when they argue that:

The term *social* justice is used rather than simply justice to show that it is more than a matter of individual fairness (although that too is very important); rather, it is a matter of understanding how social processes and institutions systematically combine to produce unfair outcomes. Social justice is therefore a *sociopolitical* matter, rather than simply a matter of personal ethics. It reflects the *social* nature of social work and its links with wider social and political issues.

(Thompson and Thompson, 2016, p. 247)

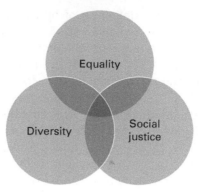

Figure 1.1 Equality, diversity and social justice

When it comes to social justice, then, social work is in a pivotal position, in so far as the individual and collective actions of members of the profession can either challenge and undermine the processes that produce unfair outcomes (by promoting equality) or can reinforce them (for example, by basing our practice on discriminatory assumptions). It is therefore important that social work is committed to promoting social justice.

Oppression

If we recall that discrimination is the process by which differences are identified and people are treated unfairly ('less favourably' to use the technical term) because of those differences, then we can take our analysis a step further by understanding that oppression is the outcome of that unfair treatment. That is, the unfair treatment associated with discrimination has oppressive consequences for the people so affected. To develop our understanding of discrimination further we therefore need to have a reasonable grasp of the oppression it gives rise to.

It is important to note at this point that differences between this book and the work of authors who distinguish between anti-discriminatory and anti-oppressive practice are primarily semantic, rather than theoretical or ideological. In order to promote forms of practice that are genuinely emancipatory, it is necessary to address the processes of discrimination that give rise to oppression. So, whether we refer to such endeavours as anti-discriminatory or anti-oppressive practice, is in my view not a significant issue. What is significant is that we seek to reduce oppression by tackling the processes of discrimination that give rise to it.

In Chapter 2, I offer a definition of oppression which includes the idea that it involves: 'the negative and demeaning exercise of power'. Similarly, *Webster's Third New International Dictionary* uses the phrase 'unjust or cruel exercise of authority or power' in its definition of oppression. Power and oppression are therefore closely linked (Mullaly, 2009).

In order to understand oppression as a dimension of the lives of social work clients (and potential clients), it is therefore necessary to be clear about the part played by power and how it operates. This is particularly important, as power is a unifying theme across the various subsections of this chapter – it is a concept which can be seen to apply in each of the topics covered. It links together what may otherwise appear a relatively unrelated series of issues.

Where social workers, and indeed other human services professionals, come into contact with clients, power is always on the agenda; it is a basic part of how people interact in general, and especially how professionals relate to their clientele. This is very much the case in terms of the power of men in relation to women, white people in relation to black, young in relation to old, and able-bodied in relation to disabled, and so on. In addition, we must recognize the power of social workers in terms of:

● knowledge and expertise;

● access to resources;

● statutory powers; and

● influence over individuals, agencies and so on.

Power is an aspect of the relationship between social workers and their clients – in addition to the social divisions which go to make up the social structure (Payne, 2006). This raises two sets of potential problems:

1 The social worker's power can be used in an oppressive way – that is, it can be abused (Thompson, 2007).

2 The social worker may not be sufficiently sensitive to issues of power/ powerlessness and oppression as they relate to clients in terms of their social location – gender, race, age and so on.

Anti-discriminatory practice therefore needs to be very sensitive to issues of power, and not simply in relation to the main areas of discrimination discussed in this book.

Voice of experience 1.2

It worried me quite a bit when I was a student, what with all this talk of the power of the social worker and the potential for oppression. But I was lucky that when I first qualified I had a line manager who was really good at helping me understand that, as long as I was true to my values and was alert to what was going on around me, I would be in a strong position to deal with the challenges involved. *Sam, a social worker in a youth justice service*

Oppression is also significant in relation to identity (Parekh, 2008). The traditional view of identity as a narrow, psychological issue is increasingly being challenged as sociological and political aspects of identity are receiving greater attention (Pullen, Beech and Sims, 2007). And oppression is an important factor in understanding this wider view of identity formation. Woodward challenges the narrowness of conventional views of identity when she argues that:

> identities are forged through the marking of difference. This marking of difference takes place both through the symbolic systems of representation, and through forms of social exclusion. Identity, then, is not the opposite of, but depends on, difference. In social relations, these forms of symbolic and social difference are established, at least in part, through the operation of what are called classificatory systems. A classificatory system applies a principle of difference to a population in such a way as to be able to divide them and all their characteristics into at least two, opposing groups – us/them (e.g. Serb/Croat); self/other.
>
> (Woodward, 1997, p. 29)

It follows, then, that it is important for social work education and practice (particularly in relation to assessment, for example) to take on board this broader conception of identity. An individual's identity will owe much to his or her social location and thus possible or actual experiences of discrimination and oppression.

Social workers have at times been criticized for taking too narrow and individualistic an approach, and thus failing to appreciate wider social patterns (Mills, 1970). Social workers who seek to develop anti-discriminatory practice need not only to move beyond the micro level of the individual level to understand the macro level of the sociopolitical, but also to appreciate how the sociopolitical domain has a major impact on the personal and subjective. Who I am is not just a matter of my unique and personal life-world, it is also a matter of my social location and to what extent and in what ways I may experience oppression. As Lawler (2008) puts it: 'identity needs to be understood not as belonging "within" the individual, but as produced between persons and within social relations' (p. 8).

The various forms of oppression – be it sexism, racism, disablism, heterosexism, sectarianism or internal colonialism and so on – can be seen to have a potential impact on identity in terms of:

● alienation, isolation, marginalization;

● economic position and life chances;

● confidence and self-esteem; and

● social expectations, career opportunities and so on.

The links between identity and oppression are significant, although an analysis which does justice to these issues is far beyond the scope of a more generalized, introductory text such as this. The basic linkages should none the less be borne in mind when considering the various sources of oppression discussed below.

Practice focus 1.2

Tim had many years' experience as an unqualified worker before commencing his professional training. That experience, though, was entirely in a fieldwork team where he dealt exclusively with individuals and families on a casework basis. On the first placement of his course, however, he worked on a community development project where, for the first time, he was able to see the shared problems, the commonalities of poverty, deprivation, racism and so on. With the help of his practice teacher he was able to understand the structural dimension of social problems and to appreciate the need to go beyond individual or family problems.

One further aspect of oppression I wish to consider is that of its complex, multifaceted nature. There can be no simple or crude model of oppression, and especially no spurious 'hierarchy of oppressions' (that is, no ranking of one form of discrimination as being somehow more significant or more important than the others). As we have noted, oppression is a dimension, or outcome, of a power relationship, specifically a relationship premised on discrimination. Such relationships are, of course, diverse and many sided, forming an intricate web of social patterns and interactions. To reduce this to a simplistic, one-dimensional model of oppression as the evil or unenlightened behaviour and attitudes of certain social groups (men, white people and so on) is a form of crude 'reductionism', in the sense that it reduces a complex, highly variable situation to the status of a monolithic, undifferentiated concept (Sibeon, 2004; Thompson, 2000a). It is to the significance of this that we now turn.

Multiple oppressions

There are many texts available which concentrate on a particular aspect of anti-discriminatory practice, whether this be anti-racism (Williams and Johnson, 2010), anti-ageism (S. Thompson, 2005) and so on. This book, however, is not intended simply as an introduction to each of the discrete areas. There is an underlying thread of 'multiple oppression', the inter-weaving of various sources and forms of oppression.

Discrimination and the oppression it gives rise to are presented as aspects of the divisive nature of social structure – reflections of such social divisions as class, race, gender, age, disability, sexuality, language group, religion and sexual identity. These are dimensions of our social location (where and how we fit into society), and so we need to understand them as a whole – facets of an overall edifice of power and dominance, rather than separate or discrete entities. To use an existentialist term, they are 'dimensions of our lived experience'.

Race, class, gender and so on tend to be separated out for analytical purposes, but they are, of course, not entirely separate processes; they occur simultaneously and affect people in combination. They are related dimensions of our complex existence, rather than discrete entities.

There is a need for a wider analysis which goes beyond class, race and gender to include marginalization on the grounds of age, disability, sexuality and other such 'social divisions'. What is called for is an integrated approach, a holistic perspective which recognizes the reality of multiple oppressions which seeks to concentrate on the commonalities and shared aspects of alienation, marginalization and discrimination. In short, political energies should be directed towards challenging oppression in its various forms, rather than in-fighting between different anti-discrimination interest groups.

This is, of course, more easily said than done, but the argument does have implications for social work policy and practice. The notion of an integrated analysis is a central one to this book, as my focus will be very clearly on the conception of anti-discriminatory practice as a unitary whole (rather than simply the sum total of anti-sexism plus anti-racism plus anti-ageism and so on). It has to be recognized that the combination of oppressions and their interaction is a complex, intricate and relatively under-researched area, but one which none the less needs to be addressed (see *Promoting Equality*). Discrimination and oppression are multifaceted phenomena, and so it is important to gain an understanding of both the common themes across areas and the key differences between them (see Chapter 9).

Practice focus 1.3

Sue was keen to work in an anti-discriminatory way in assessing Mrs Desai's needs under the NHS and Community Care Act 1990 and therefore paid close attention to Mrs Desai's cultural background and needs and her experiences of racism. However, it was only in a subsequent supervision session that she realized that her anti-discriminatory focus had been one-dimensional. That is, she had neglected to consider issues of gender and sexism or, indeed, the profound effects of ageism on Mrs Desai. Sue was fortunate in having a team leader who had a good understanding of anti-discriminatory issues, and who was able to help her develop her understanding and skills in this demanding aspect of practice.

Avoiding medicalization

In order to foster equality, diversity and social justice, there are various things that we need to do. Chief among these is the need to avoid 'medicalization' – that is, the process of translating personal and social problems into medical matters. This has the effect of 'pathologizing' people and is a form of reductionism – which once again involves reducing a complex, multidimensional situation to a simple matter of 'illness' or 'disorder'. Mental health issues are a good example of this.

People who are deemed to be mentally disordered often encounter a negative response, even to the point of outright hostility, from the community at large. However, it is often the case that the response of professionals can also be experienced as oppressive. This is due, in no small part, to the tendency to view issues of mental disorder in terms of a medical model – that is, to adopt a 'medicalized' approach. Such an approach has been criticized by many (for example, Bentall, 2004, 2010; Crossley, 2006; Gambrill, 2005; Tew 2011; see also my *Promoting Equality*) for its narrow and distorted perspective which presents moral, social and political matters as medical problems and therefore clearly located within the domain of the medical profession (and the pharmaceutical industry).

The critique of the medical model is not a new idea. For example, as long ago as 1986, Busfield described Szasz's views on this issue (which themselves date back to the 1960s) in the following terms:

> The notion of mental illness is, Szasz claims, but a metaphor for what should, more accurately, be called 'problems in living', for except for the organic mental illnesses (those with identifiable physical causes) which would be better thought of as brain diseases, what is termed mental illness mystifies what is in fact a moral judgement, for the term illness suggests a scientific and objective assessment of sickness based on identifiable physical pathology. On the contrary it is a moral judgement and should be recognized as such.
>
> (Busfield, 1986, p. 86)

Translating moral issues into medical ones has two implications which are particularly relevant to anti-discriminatory practice:

1 *Power* The 'medicalization' of mental disorder gives considerable power to members of the medical profession and the administrative, technical and professional structures of which they form a part.

2 *Stereotypes* The classification system inherent in the medical model can be seen to have the effect of producing stereotypes of people said to be suffering from 'mental illness'. It concentrates on generalities at the expense of specifics (Pickering, 2001).

These are both key aspects of the process of discrimination and the oppression that results. We therefore need to look carefully at their impact on clients and systems of service delivery.

Key point 1.2

Attaching a stigmatizing label to someone can do a great deal of harm. It is therefore essential that we look at situations holistically, taking account of the wider issues, rather than rely on a medical label that does not do justice to the complexities involved.

The power of the medical profession to define and control deviance is a long-established one which is not commonly challenged within social work practice on a day-to-day basis. This power base and its influence on social work thinking and practice can act as a significant obstruction to the development of a social work of empowerment. This applies in a number of ways – for example:

1 As Chamberlin comments:

> once a person is labelled 'mentally ill', he or she loses fundamental rights that everyone else takes for granted. In fact, most so-called anti-stigma campaigns are run by the very people and organizations that control and support the process of diagnosis and treatment. ... Once a person has been defined as mentally ill, his or her own decision-making ability is called into question, and therefore, his or her protests are often discredited or, even worse, labelled one more 'symptom' of his or her illness.
>
> (Chamberlin, 2006, p. xi)

2 Medical discourse separates the individual's experience of pain or distress from the wider social context which underpins it. Thus the emphasis is on 'treating' individuals rather than tackling the underlying sources of distress. As Bentall argues:

> *We should abandon psychiatric diagnoses altogether and instead try to explain and understand the actual experiences and behaviours of psychotic people.* By such experiences and behaviours I mean the kinds of things that psychiatrists describe as symptoms, but which might be better labelled complaints, such as hallucinations, delusions and disordered speech. I will argue that, once these complaints have been explained, there is no ghostly disease remaining that also requires an explanation. Complaints are all there is.
>
> (Bentall, 2004, p. 141)

I would want to make sure that the explanation of these complaints also includes reference to wider sociopolitical factors, and is not just limited to psychological explanations (which would amount to replacing one form of reductionism with another).

Both these points illustrate the danger of 'blaming the victim' (Ryan, 1988) by reducing a complex web of psychological, social, moral, political and economic factors to a simple pathology 'within' the individual.

These two examples relate both to power and to the individual, but in different ways. In the first, the personal power of the individual is denied and, in the second, the effects of wider processes and structures are translated into individual pathology. In both cases the individual is disempowered.

Similar issues apply to the process of stereotyping. Medicine claims to be an objective science and therefore seeks to establish clear and explicit diagnostic categories. And, of course, when categories are being applied to people, the danger of stereotyping is one to be wary of.

This applies particularly to the diagnostic label of 'schizophrenia' which is a much disputed concept. It has been criticized by many as a vague 'catch-all' which covers a broad range of problems (see, for example, Bentall, 2004; Boyle, 2002). Applying labels to people on the basis of a dubious scientific objectivity is a process which has distinctly oppressive connotations. There is a clear danger of setting up stereotypical expectations which have profoundly negative and discriminatory implications.

It is evident, therefore, that an uncritical approach to mental health social work which adopts the tenets of the medical model is not conducive to anti-discriminatory practice. What is called for is an approach which is more holistic, in so far as it is more attuned to cultural and structural factors and does not stop short at the individual level.

As we shall see in Chapter 2, cultural factors are important in terms of shared meanings and values – the context in which the supposedly 'schizophrenic' behaviour can be rendered intelligible (Crossley, 2006). That is, we cannot assume, as conventional psychiatry does, that 'mad' behaviour is meaningless and without foundation. An anti-discriminatory approach would be less dismissive and would be more attuned to Laing's

> long struggle to show that those labelled 'schizophrenic' are coherent in their agony – that their turns of phrase, silences, behaviour and hallucinations make a certain sense, given some dispassionate knowledge of the relationships within which they are located.
>
> (Ticktin, 1989, p. 4)

Structural factors are also very relevant. Consider, for example, the links between gender and mental health (Fawcett and Karban, 2005) or race and mental health (Fernando, 2010). But even beyond this, the medical model can itself be seen as a generalized vehicle of oppression. As Fernando comments:

> When present-day psychiatrists ... diagnose schizophrenia, in effect they stigmatize – although admittedly many do not realize it. So the clear message is that to get rid of stigma we need to get rid of the genetic-biomedical model of mental illness.
>
> (Fernando, 2010, p. 39)

Thornicroft (2006) describes in detail the various ways in which people with mental health problems can be stigmatized and discriminated against, but his work is presented in the language of medicine and pathology. A truly anti-discriminatory approach to mental health issues would need to go beyond such an uncritical acceptance of a medical model of mental distress.

Clearly, this view raises a number of issues which merit much more attention than I am able to devote to them here. None the less, I hope my main point is clear, namely that the medical model, with its individualist and pathologizing focus has a discriminatory and oppressive impact, and is therefore not an adequate basis for anti-discriminatory social work practice.

It is also worth emphasizing that, while I have used mental health as an example of the problematic adoption of a medicalized perspective on life problems, this is not the only area of social work to which it applies. As we shall see in later chapters, it is also a problematic feature of how other groups are treated by the helping professions – older people and disabled people, for example. It is a common feature of discrimination.

Conclusion

This is the first of two chapters geared towards laying down the foundations of a theoretical understanding of discrimination on the premise that an approach that lacks such understanding is likely to be, at best, an ineffective one and, at worst, counterproductive (Thompson, 2010). It has provided an overview of such key concepts as discrimination, equality, diversity, social justice, oppression and medicalization. We are now ready to move on to explore the theory base more fully in order to take further our understanding of the complex issues involved in developing approaches to practice that are truly emancipatory – that is, which help us to tackle discrimination and oppression.

Food for thought

- What practical steps can be taken to promote equality?
- Why is it important to 'value diversity'?

- In what ways can social work be seen as part of a commitment to social justice?

- Why is it important to avoid 'medicalizing' personal and social problems?

Further resources

Promoting Equality (Thompson, 2011a) develops many aspects of the discussion in this chapter. Thompson (2007) focuses in particular on issues relating to power and empowerment. Beyond my own work there is a wealth of relevant literature that can be drawn upon to take our knowledge and understanding further – for example, Baxter (*Managing Diversity and Inequality in Health Care*, 2001) on diversity; Mullaly (*Challenging Oppression and Confronting Privilege*, 2009) on oppression; and Cohen and Timini (*Liberatory Psychiatry: Philosophy, Politics and Mental Health*, 2008) and Kirk, Gomory and Cohen (*Mad Science: Psychiatry, Coercion, Diagnosis, and Drugs*, 2015) on medicalization. Barry (*Why Social Justice Matters*, 2005) is a very helpful text in relation to social justice – all social workers should read this book. Hills (*Good Times, Bad Times: The Welfare Myth of Them and Us*, 2015) is also an important contribution to our understanding.

CHAPTER 2

THE THEORY BASE

CHAPTER OVERVIEW

In this chapter you will:

- Learn about the significance of the various ways in which society divides people into groups or categories (class, gender and so on)
- Explore a theoretical model (PCS analysis) which emphasizes the importance of understanding the personal, cultural and structural aspects of discrimination and the interrelationships across the three
- Appreciate how discrimination can arise in complex ways that are not simply matters of personal prejudice and not necessarily intentional

Introduction

Social work theory derives from a wide range of sources although, traditionally, the social work literature owes much to social science thinking. In particular, the theory base I am outlining here draws heavily on sociology and social psychology and is underpinned by insights drawn from existentialism (Thompson, 2010).

This is not of course primarily a theoretical text – the major focus is on anti-discriminatory *practice*. But, an understanding of the underlying conceptual framework, and the themes and concepts of which it consists, is necessary to ensure that such practice is based on intelligent and informed debate, rather than dogma, fad or ignorance. Indeed, discrimination and oppression as a field of study has been prone to more than its fair share of dogma and oversimplification over the years (see Thompson, 2009b, for a critique).

I shall therefore present an exposition of some of the key themes and issues and sketch out some of the linkages between the theoretical concepts and the social work concerns they are intended to illuminate. This will, of course, be a far from comprehensive account – a text of this size devoted entirely to such issues would still barely do justice to the complexity and scope of the subject matter (see *Promoting Equality* for a more detailed exposition of the theory base). This chapter is therefore very much an introductory exploration of the theory base. It is a beginning which, I hope, will have the effect of both equipping and motivating the reader to build on these foundations through further reading, discussion and above all, relating such theory to practice.

Social divisions and social structure

Societies are not, of course, simply amorphous masses of people. A society comprises a diverse range of people and is therefore characterized by differentiation – people are categorized according to social divisions such as class and gender. These divisions then form the basis of the social structure – the 'network' of social relationships, institutions and groupings – which plays such an important role in the distribution of power, status and opportunities.

It has long been recognized that people can be 'located' within the social structure in terms of the intersection of different social divisions (Payne, 2006). That is, who we are depends to a large extent on how and where we fit into society. And this, in turn, depends on the complex web of social divisions or social 'strata' (hence the term 'stratification'). These strata are many and varied, but the emphasis here will be on the major social divisions, those of class (Roberts, 2011), gender (Gruber and Stefanov, 2002), race/ethnicity (Back and Solomos, 2009), age (S. Thompson, 2005) disability (Swain et al., 2014), sexuality (Carabine, 2004a, b) and religion (Moss, 2005). This is not to deny the importance or relevance of other social divisions, such as linguistic group, region or mental status. It is simply a matter of having to be realistic in restricting the scope of the analysis for reasons of space.

Let us look briefly at each of these dimensions of the social structure before considering their significance for social work.

Class

There is a long-standing major debate within sociology concerning the definition of class (Roberts, 2011). There are those who, following Marx, define class in relation to ownership or control of the means of production (specifically, the means of producing wealth – land, factories, machinery and so on). There are others, who, following Weber, relate class to 'relations of exchange' (that is, buying power) rather than relations of production. (See Giddens, 2009, for an overview of these issues and Giddens, 1971, for a fuller discussion.)

Within social work the term tends to be used loosely, in a broadly Weberian sense, to indicate different levels of economic power. Low class position (equals low economic power due to low pay or reliance on benefits) is associated with poverty, poor-quality housing, poor health and a general lack of opportunity. Dobelniece highlights the consequences of living in poverty:

> Poor people get less of everything that is considered important and necessary for a decent life, that is, less money, food, clothing, shelter. The deprivation experienced by poor people is pervasive. Children brought up in poverty are more likely to fail in school, to drop out of school. They are more likely to develop mental health problems, are more susceptible to chronic illnesses, and are less likely to be covered by health insurance. They are more likely to lose jobs and to drop out of the labour force. They are more likely to experience hostility and distrust. They are less likely to participate in meaningful groups and associations. As the ultimate deprivation, they are likely to die at a younger age.
>
> (Dobelniece, 1998, pp. 5–6)

Hills (2015) points out that the UK is one of the six most unequal countries in the industrialized world. He also informs us that this inequality has been increasing, with people at the lower levels of the income spectrum receiving an increasingly lower proportion of the overall wealth available. The relationship between class, poverty and social work is therefore a very significant one (Garrett, 2002).

Gender

There are distinct and relatively fixed biological differences between men and women. These are *sex* differences. However, when we ascribe particular social significance to these differences, and allot roles accordingly, they become *gender* differences. That is, it becomes a matter of social construction rather than biological determination (Burr, 2003).

Boys and girls are socialized into differential patterns of behaviour, interaction, thought, language and emotional response. Different roles are assigned, according to gender, and so differential sets of expectations are established. These expectations are constantly reinforced through social interaction and the influence of the media, the education system and so on. Where people deviate from these gender expectations, sanctions are applied – boys who stray into feminine territory are labelled 'cissy' or 'effeminate' while girls who transgress are seen as 'butch' or a 'tomboy'. These childhood patterns become deeply ingrained and persist through to adulthood.

Gender expectations can also produce a situation whereby the same characteristic can be interpreted differently according to whether it applies to a man or a woman. For example, assertiveness in men can be seen as strength of character, whereas in women it can be seen as bossiness (Thompson, 2015a). The cycle is complete when biological sex differences are used to justify or 'legitimate' the inequalities inherent in social differences based on gender. This is an important point and so this link between the biological and the social will feature again below in the discussion of ideology.

Race and ethnicity

'Race', like sex, is often assumed to be a biological matter, but this is a misleading assumption to make. Blackburn argues that the assumed biological basis of 'race' is a common fallacy and goes on to point out that: 'biologically, there is one race – the human race – in its modest variety and overwhelming commonality' (2000, p. 19). Similarly, Muldoon, in discussing the history of slavery, argues that:

> The relationship between slave and master was fixed by a biological imperative. It was a law of nature that could not be repealed. The medieval notion that humanity was one and that humankind had the same capacity for transformation was replaced by a pseudoscientific view that people existed as biologically different races, the mental and moral capacities of which were fixed for all time.
>
> (Muldoon, 2000, p. 92)

It is partly for this reason that the term 'race' often has the word 'ethnicity' attached to it – to emphasize that it refers to a social grouping rather than a biological one. That is, it is the equivalent of gender rather than sex. For the same reason, many authors consistently place inverted commas around the word ('race') in order to indicate that it is not being used in its literal, (pseudo-)biological sense.

Jivraj and Simpson helpfully explain the fluid and rather indeterminate nature of ethnicity when they point out that:

> Measuring ethnicity is fraught with difficulty because researchers try to reduce a subjective and dynamic concept to a categorization that is

meaningful to individuals and, at the same time, manageable in data analysis. Bulmer (2010) suggests an ethnic group is a collectivity within a large population with shared identity defined by kinship, religion, language, shared territory, nationality or physical appearance. The importance of these dimensions in what shapes ethnic identity will vary from person to person. Moreover, the differences become blurred in multicultural societies such as Britain, where living in diverse areas has meant minority groups have borrowed from one another and the majority culture to form new identities. This makes it more difficult than ever to distinguish meaningful categories (Neal et al., 2013).

(Jivraj and Simpson, 2015, p. 2)

We need to recognize, then, that ethnicity is not a simple or straightforward matter, but it is none the less a very important issue, as a person's identity is strongly linked to their ethnicity and undermining a person's sense of identity can create a lot of ill feeling and do a lot of harm.

Voice of experience 2.1

I am White, British and have lived in a rural part of the UK all my life, and I suppose I have always taken my ethnicity for granted. But when I did a placement in a city area, where there were people from a wide range of backgrounds, I was amazed at just how many differences there were and just how important those differences are to people. It taught me not to take ethnicity for granted ever again.
Steve, a mental health social worker

Race is therefore a socially constructed way of categorizing people on the basis of assumed biological differences (Malik, 2008). As with socially constructed gender distinctions, the notion of race entails:

- *Inherent inequalities*   Racial categorization involves not only difference but also implies relations of superiority/inferiority. This is the basis of racism (see Chapter 4).

- *Biological legitimation*   The biological aspect of this social division is used as a justification for discrimination and inequality.

Some people might argue that, because it does not have a biological basis, race does not exist. It does exist, but it is a social construction, rather than a biological entity. Social constructions are very real. For example, the law is a social construction and, as Malik (2008) points out, so too is money.

Age

The problems associated with sexism and racism have long been recognized and are relatively well documented. Discrimination on the grounds of age, or 'ageism', as it has become known, is a relatively new addition to anti-discriminatory discourse. One long-standing definition of ageism describes it in the following terms: 'Ageism means unwarranted application of negative stereotypes to older people' (Fennell, Phillipson and Evers, 1988, p. 97). As we shall see in Chapter 5, old age is strongly associated with notions of frailty, mental and physical debility and dependency. This association is greatly exaggerated by common (mis)conceptions about the nature of old age and the incidence of problems. This tendency to devalue older people and overemphasize the negative aspects of later life is characteristic of ageism (Powell, 2006). The distribution of power, status and opportunities is therefore dependent upon not only class, race and gender but also age. Age is therefore an important social division, a significant dimension of the social structure. The main focus of anti-ageism is old age, but when we consider that very similar issues apply to children (S. Thompson, 2005), the impact of ageism takes on additional significance. Indeed, we could go beyond the definition of Fennell et al. (1988) of ageism to include children: 'discrimination against any individual or group on the basis of age'.

Disability

Disability is a concept that distinguishes a certain proportion of the population (those with some degree of physical impairment) from the 'able-bodied' majority. Again, this is not simply a biological/physiological matter but has major social implications. By defining disability as primarily a physiological matter, the issues are personalized, individualized and medicalized. In this way the social and political dimensions are overlooked (Barnes and Mercer, 2010).

Proponents of what has come to be known as a social model of disability have argued that traditional, individualized approaches to disability mask the inherent marginalization and dehumanization involved in attitudes and policies in relation to people with disabilities (Oliver, 2009). The biological level is used as a means of legitimating unequal power relations at the social and political levels. Disablism is the term used to describe the oppression and discrimination implicit in this situation – the social division of disability.

Practice focus 2.1

Pearlene was an experienced social worker whose work had mainly been in the field of mental health. However, her new post was in a disability team. As part of her induction programme she attended a meeting of the local disability forum. This was to be a significant event for her as she was amazed to see how much anger there was against local service providers and how patronized the disabled people at the forum felt by medically oriented social work and nursing staff. She realized that her common-sense views of disability and disabled people's needs would have to be reconsidered.

Sexuality

There are, of course, different categories of sexuality (heterosexual or 'straight'; gay; lesbian; bisexual and so on), but these are not accorded equal status. To belong to a minority group in terms of sexuality is to find oneself open to significant discrimination. Sadly, despite major steps forward as a result of the gay liberation movement, the problem of discrimination on the grounds of sexuality (or sexual identity or orientation) remains of major proportions (Moon, 2008). At times this can have important implications for social work and we will explore these in Chapter 7.

Sexuality is another example of a complex psychosocial phenomenon (that is, one that is shaped in large part by a combination of psychological and sociological factors) that is often reduced to a biological explanation. For example, the diversity of forms of sexuality is often dismissed as 'unnatural', an aberration from the assumed biological norm of a single 'natural' sexuality – that is, heterosexuality.

Religion

To belong to a particular faith community is to be located within the social structure in terms of religion. Just like ethnicity, gender or age, religion divides people into groups that can then be discriminated against by other (usually more powerful) groups (other religions, sects or non-religious groups). This is a very complex field of study, but one which at times has wide-ranging implications for social work. It is for this reason that Chapter 8 will explore why issues of religious affiliation are very significant in general and in relation to discrimination in particular.

In some ways religious discrimination overlaps (and interacts) with racial discrimination, but there are also important issues to consider that relate specifically to religious faith.

The individualistic, largely psychodynamic focus of traditional social work has been criticized for its failure to take account of the social dimension. From this critique, systems theory developed, with its explicit emphasis on social systems. This, in turn, was subsequently criticized for ignoring the importance of conflict, structure and social divisions and for being dehumanizing in its language and approach (Thompson, 1992). Social work theory has now progressed to a level of sophistication at which the part played by social divisions and sociopolitical factors is receiving increasing attention. However, what is needed is a conceptual framework that will enable us to develop a clearer understanding of how the problems social workers and their clients face can be located in this wider sociological context. What I shall refer to as PCS analysis can take us some considerable way towards this, and so it is to this topic that we shall now turn.

PCS analysis

In order to understand how inequalities and discrimination feature in the social circumstances of clients, and in the interactions between clients and social work professionals (and indeed in the lives of social workers themselves who can so easily be discriminated against), it is helpful to analyse the situation in terms of three levels. These three levels (**P**, **C** and **S**) are closely interlinked and constantly interact with one another (see Figure 2.1).

P refers to the personal or psychological; it is the individual level of thoughts, feelings, attitudes and actions. It also refers to practice, individual workers interacting with individual clients, and prejudice, the inflexibility of mind which stands in the way of fair and non-judgemental practice. Our thoughts, feelings and attitudes about particular groups in society will, to a certain degree at least, be shaped by our experiences at a personal level.

C refers to the cultural level of shared ways of seeing, thinking and doing. It relates to the commonalities – values and patterns of thought and behaviour, an assumed consensus about what is right and what is normal; it produces conformity to social norms, and comic humour acts

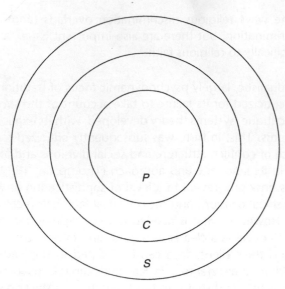

Figure 2.1 PCS analysis

as a vehicle for transmitting and reinforcing this culture. It is therefore primarily a matter of shared meanings. It includes conventional notions of culture, such as religion, belief systems and nationality, but goes beyond these. The cultural level is a complex web of taken-for-granted assumptions or 'unwritten rules'. Culture is very influential in determining what is perceived as 'normal' in any given set of circumstances.

S refers to the structural level, the network of social divisions and the power relations that are so closely associated with them; it also relates to the ways in which oppression and discrimination are 'institutionalized' (firmly established through patterns of thought, language and behaviour) and thus 'sewn in' to the fabric of society. It denotes the wider level of social forces, the sociopolitical dimension of interlocking patterns of power and influence.

The **P** level is, as Figure 2.1 illustrates, embedded within the cultural or **C** level – that is, the **C** level forms the context in which our personal experience occurs. Our thoughts, actions, attitudes and feelings are to a certain extent unique and individualized, but we must also recognize the powerful role of culture in forming our opinions, guiding our actions and so on.

The **C** level represents the interests and the influence of society as reflected in the social values and cultural norms we internalize via the process of socialization – for example, manners, etiquette and rituals (such as to how to behave towards someone when it is their birthday or they have just become engaged). In a classic work of sociology Peter Berger captures this point well:

> Only an understanding of internalization makes sense of the incredible fact that most external controls work most of the time for most of the people in a society. Society not only controls our movements, but shapes our identity, our thoughts and our emotions. The structures of society become the structure of our own consciousness. Society does not stop at the surface of our skins. Society penetrates us as much as it envelops us.
>
> (Berger, 1966, p. 140)

This passage is particularly relevant to the cultural influence of forms of discrimination on individual consciousness. It lays the foundations for understanding the various forms of discrimination not simply as personal prejudice (the **P** level) but, more realistically, the discriminatory and oppressive culture base manifesting itself in and through individual thought and action. It is therefore a more complex situation involving the interaction of the **P** and **C** levels.

Humour is an example of how a discriminatory culture can subtly but powerfully influence individual thoughts and actions. For example, racist jokes can be seen as a vehicle for reinforcing and legitimating notions of racial superiority. The fact that humour is so highly valued as a social quality means that it is both a highly potent influence and relatively well defended from attack. Comments such as 'it's only a joke' or 'it's only a bit of fun' act as effective defences and help to maintain the discriminatory power of humour. This is not to say that humour is necessarily discriminatory – far from it – but, where it does have oppressive potential, we need to be wary of allowing ourselves to be seduced by it.

To say that the **P** level is embedded within the **C** level is not to suggest that the thoughts and actions of individuals are simply a 'reflection' of society or culture. PCS analysis is not deterministic; it does not imply that culture 'causes' our actions, but rather that individual behaviour has to be understood in the wider cultural context.

But even this cultural context needs to be understood in terms of a wider context – the structural. That is, the **C** level is embedded within the **S** level. It is no coincidence that we have the cultural and social formations that currently exist. These owe much to the structure of society – the interlocking matrix of social divisions and the power relations which maintain them. To understand the **C** level we need to relate it to the **S** level, the structure of society.

Marx argued that the economic base or 'infrastructure' conditions the 'superstructure' – that is, the political, social and cultural aspects (the **C** level). This is an argument about class, the class conflict in the economic base of capitalism. But, as was argued in Chapter 1, class is not the only structural dimension which merits our attention.

Feminists have convincingly argued the case for recognizing the importance of gender in mapping out the social structure (Richardson and Robinson, 2007), while the anti-racist movement has built on the foundations of a plea for understanding the racially structured nature of modern western societies (Williams and Johnson, 2010). These will both be discussed further in Chapters 3 and 4 respectively. The significance of age and disability as relevant dimensions of the social structure is also being increasingly recognized, as some of the discussions in this text will confirm.

Marx's analysis does not, therefore, take us far enough, but it is, none the less, a useful beginning. Indeed, I would contend that it is a grave mistake to reject the key elements of marxism – a case of throwing the baby out with the bath water. I shall return to this point in the concluding chapter.

PCS analysis shows the different levels at which discrimination operates and how these levels reinforce each other. What is also worth noting, however, is that the degree of control and impact a worker can have on tackling discrimination is also related to the three levels, as is shown in Figure 2.2.

The further away one moves from the personal level, the less impact an individual can have. It therefore becomes necessary to move beyond the personal level, not only in terms of understanding discrimination but

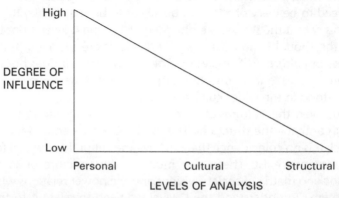

Figure 2.2 Degrees of influence

also in terms of tackling it. This involves individuals playing their part in *collectively* challenging the dominant discriminatory culture and ideology and, in so doing, playing at least a part in the undermining of the structures which support, and are supported by, that culture.

Structured inequalities and institutional discrimination

One of the advantages of using PCS analysis is that it shows the inadequacy of explanations which stop short at the individual level. For example, it is not enough to explain racism as a personal prejudice or the wicked misdeeds of a bigoted minority, such as members of extreme right-wing organizations. In fact, this more overt and openly embraced type of racial discrimination is referred to by many as 'racialism' (see, for example, Todorov, 2009) to distinguish it from the wider concept of racism. As we shall see in Chapter 4, racism can be by omission as well as commission. It is not simply a matter of prejudicial beliefs.

If we accept that we live in a society characterized by racism (in the sense that it is a society that is geared to the white majority and thus tends to systematically disadvantage ethnic minorities – see the discussion of institutional discrimination below and of institutional racism in particular in Chapter 4), then it is not surprising that racist beliefs and practices will have been learned and 'taken on board' as parts of our personalities and what Berger and Luckmann (1967) call 'the taken-for-grantedness of everyday life'. Even if we are full of good intentions in relation to anti-discriminatory practice, unless we are actively seeking to eliminate racist thoughts and actions from our day-to-day dealings, they will 'filter through' from the culture and structure into which we were socialized and which constantly seek to influence us (through the media, political propaganda and so on). It is in this sense that we cannot remain 'neutral'. As the political slogan would have it: 'if you're not part of the solution, you must be part of the problem'. That is, the tide of discrimination (the **C** and **S** levels) is so strong that, unless we actively swim against it, it is more or less inevitable that we will be carried along with it.

A key aspect of this is the need to recognize that most discrimination is unintentional – it arises because of institutionalized patterns of behaviour, assumptions and language use more frequently than through deliberate acts intended to disadvantage particular individuals or groups (although the latter are, of course, sadly not uncommon).

Tackling discrimination, then, is not simply a matter of identifying the guilty parties, the bigots and chauvinists. The reality is far more complex than this, as it needs to be recognized that – to paraphrase Edmund Burke – all that is necessary for evil to flourish is for good people to do nothing.

I have used the example of racism, but much the same can be said of the other forms of discrimination. For example, in terms of sexism, it is not simply a matter of a relatively small number of men who are overtly sexist or 'male chauvinist pigs'. Sexism subtly pervades our thoughts and actions and very often influences us in ways which we do not recognize until somebody points them out to us. (It is for this reason that 'Awareness Training' is an important prerequisite for anti-discriminatory practice – see Chapter 9.) Oppression and discrimination cannot be explained simply by reference to personal prejudice. Katz's (1978) classic notion of 'prejudice plus power' takes us in the right direction, but ultimately confuses the issue more than it clarifies it (Sibeon, 1991a). Discrimination is a reflection (and a reinforcer) of structured inequalities. The fact that we live in such a highly stratified society means that inequalities are part and parcel of the social order – there are inevitably winners and losers. Again, this is not an individual matter, as such inequalities are 'sewn in' to the fabric of society – they underpin social order. This introduces the notion of 'institutional discrimination'.

Oppression does not derive simply from individual actions or 'praxis'. It can be, and often is, built in to institutionalized patterns and organizational policies. In what has come to be seen as a classic study, Rooney (1987) gives a good example of how this operates. He describes how one local authority used to recruit its home-help staff by word of mouth. When vacancies arose, the existing (predominantly white) workforce would be asked to let people know of such vacancies. They would, of course, pass this information on to their (predominantly white) circle of friends, some of whom would then be recruited. Consequently, this form of recruitment systematically marginalized and excluded potential black staff, albeit perhaps unintentionally.

There are many aspects of social work which run this risk of institutional discrimination (the inherent sexism of some forms of family therapy, for example – see White, 2006). The concept is therefore an important part of the theory base of anti-discriminatory practice. An important point to bear in mind is that discrimination is a matter of outcomes rather than just intentions. That is, even where no discrimination is intended, if certain individuals or groups of people experience an unfair disadvantage, then discrimination has taken place and

oppression is likely to be experienced as a result of it. Unwitting discrimination can be just as damaging (if not more so) as intentional
discrimination.

One further important point to note about PCS analysis is that all three
levels can be seen to have a spiritual dimension. Holloway and Moss
(2010) are, in my view, right to emphasize the importance of recognizing
spirituality as a key part of people's lives in general and of social work in
particular. Moss and Thompson (2007) outline how an understanding of
spirituality can add further explanatory power to each of the three levels
and thereby enrich PCS analysis as a theoretical tool. They point out that
a renewed emphasis on spirituality is:

> entirely consistent with a commitment to promoting equality and valuing
> diversity. The importance of equality issues for spirituality is evidenced
> by the fact that inequality and discrimination can clearly stand in the
> way of spiritual fulfilment. The demeaning and undermining effects
> of discrimination, while at times contributing to the development
> of resilience, can have very detrimental effects on a person's self-
> esteem and overall well-being. Indeed, social justice can be seen as an
> important value underpinning both the equality agenda and approaches
> to spirituality that recognize the importance of 'connectedness' – that is,
> of what Heidegger (1962) called 'being-in-the-world'.
>
> (Moss and Thompson, 2007, p. 6)

In considering the use of PCS analysis as a way of understanding the complexities of discrimination and oppression, we should therefore make sure
that we do not lose sight of the significance of spirituality (see Moss,
2005; Thompson, 2010, Chapter 13).

PCS analysis: a note of caution

Since I first introduced PCS analysis in the first edition of this book and
developed it in other publications (*Promoting Equality*, for example), it has
become very well established and widely used. While this can clearly be
seen as a positive development, it has left me with five concerns:

1 In my role as an external examiner at a number of universities I have
   come across many examples of students simply referring to PCS analysis without showing any real understanding of it or how it can be used.
   It is as if it has become a 'mantra' to be uttered, rather than an

analytical framework that can help us make sense of the complexities of discrimination and oppression. I am concerned to ensure that it should not be used in an unthinking or uncritical way. It should be used as a basis of critically reflective practice, not as an alternative to it. Critically reflective practice will be discussed in Chapter 9.

2   I have encountered examples of PCS analysis being distorted and used inappropriately. For example, one group of participants on a training course I ran told me that a trainer on a previous course had presented PCS analysis to them (without acknowledging its source) and had argued that, because racism exists at a structural and cultural level, then white people in this country *must* be racist at a personal level. This represents a gross distortion of PCS analysis, as it conflates the different levels. Personal racism and cultural and structural forms of racism are very different entities. Although they can be interrelated, it would be a grave mistake to equate them. Care should therefore be taken to ensure that the complexities of PCS analysis are appreciated and not allowed to form the basis of a reductionist approach.

3   Many authors have misrepresented PCS analysis by describing the **S** level as social, rather than structural. This is unfortunate as it fails to reflect the sociological basis of PCS analysis in which all three levels – personal, cultural and structural – are *social* in nature. It is therefore a significant mistake to refer to the **S** level as social as if to imply that the personal and cultural levels are not also social.

4   Some authors have referred to PCS analysis as an example of systems theory. However, while there are some superficial resemblances, PCS analysis is significantly different from systems theory and is rooted in existentialist thought (see Thompson, 2010).

5   It has been suggested to me that PCS analysis does not include a community dimension and should perhaps be extended to include the community 'level'. However, as I see it, PCS analysis is a conceptual tool that can be applied at any form of intervention, whether casework, groupwork or community work. The community is a place where personal, cultural and structural issues will all feature (see *Promoting Equality* for a discussion of the double dialectic that operates in relation to **P**, **C** and **S**), and so it is best to understand the community as a potential site of discrimination, rather than a conceptual level at which discrimination operates. It is therefore not correct to say that PCS analysis neglects the community dimension.

Key point 2.1

Discrimination is a complex matter. It operates at personal, cultural and structural levels and these levels interact and influence one another. It can be misleading and potentially dangerous to focus on one of the levels without considering the other two (and their interactions).

Ideology: the power of ideas

An ideology is a set of ideas which are associated with a particular set of social arrangements. The ideology has the effect of 'legitimating the status quo' and thus justifies, protects and reinforces those social arrangements and the power relationships inherent within them. For example, patriarchal ideology promotes traditional notions of the respective roles of men and women and strongly discourages any deviation from these. The power interests inherent in patriarchy are therefore well served by the ideology of patriarchy. In short, the ideas base safeguards the power base. In fact, this is what characterizes ideology – the power of ideas operating in the interests of power relations:

> Ideology refers to the power of ideas to maintain existing structures and social relations. For example, patriarchal ideology (patriarchy means 'the law of the father' – that is, male dominance) serves to maintain existing power relations between men and women by presenting gender roles as natural and inevitable (despite the considerable evidence to the contrary). Ideology is closely linked to power relations because it is largely through the role of ideology that power is exercised. That is, the subtle, often unquestioned, workings of ideology can be far more effective in maintaining power structures than the overt and explicit use of power, for example through force or coercion.
>
> (Thompson, 2000b, p. 56)

There are various ideologies at work in society, but it tends to be the ideas of powerful groups which become dominant or, to quote the marxist dictum: 'The ideas of the ruling class are, in every age, the ruling ideas' (quoted in Bottomore and Rubel, 1963, p. 93). The ideologies of capitalism, patriarchy and imperialism are examples of such dominant ideologies.

Ideology can be seen to operate in a number of ways – that is, a number of 'ideological devices' can be identified. The setting up of 'norms' is an important part of this. An ideology will establish what is 'normal' and, therefore, by extension, what is 'abnormal'. Ideology therefore defines deviance. 'Norm', however, is an ambiguous concept, in so far as it can refer to a statistical norm, a quantitative measure. For example, heterosexuality can be seen to be 'normal' in so far as the majority of people are heterosexual. However, 'norm' can also be used in an idealized sense to reflect what 'ought to be' – that is, an ideological norm. It is a common ideological device for the two types of norm to be conflated – for an ideological norm to masquerade as a statistical norm. For example, the ideological norm of the nuclear family is often presented as if it were a statistical norm whereas, in fact, only 21 per cent of households follow the nuclear family pattern of biological parents with their dependent children (Beaumont, 2011).

Another very common primary device is that of presenting particular goals or values as 'natural'. The use of the term 'natural' is a very powerful way of gaining approval – it is a form of legitimation (that is, it makes the things so described sound right and proper and any deviation from this as 'abnormal'). To describe, for example, the traditional male role of breadwinner as 'natural' adds a false, pseudo-biological air of legitimacy. This is a particularly significant device in terms of the ideological justification of oppression. Racism is premised on the false notion of biological/natural racial categories, sexism on the reduction of social gender roles to biological sex roles. Similarly, disablism hinges on a medical (hence biological/natural) model of disability (Oliver, Sapey and Thomas, 2012) and there is an almost direct parallel here with ageism. Indeed, the masking of the economic and sociopolitical dimensions (of old age) under the guise of a biological or natural decline is an ideological device, parallel with the 'biology is destiny' axiom of sexism and the 'racial superiority' fallacy of imperialism.

Practice focus 2.2

Phillippa was the head of care at a large residential school where she was charged with implementing the organization's equal opportunities policy. However, she found considerable resistance on the part of many staff. After months of trying to persuade her colleagues of the value of challenging discrimination, she began to recognize a pattern, a set of common themes that she kept encountering. She realized that biology was the reason commonly given for not promoting equality. Race, gender and so on were all seen as biological differences and therefore natural and not open to change. Phillippa therefore decided that she would need to think of ways of convincing them of the flaws in their argument, ways of showing them that biology was only one factor in a very complex situation.

The terms 'normal' and 'natural' both tend to have strong ideological overtones, and so we should be very careful in using them and sensitize ourselves to their use by other people. The logic of discrimination is perpetuated by ideology, and so we should be very wary of these common ideological devices. Ideology refers to both the set of ideas which 'serve as weapons of social interests' (Berger and Luckmann, 1967, p. 18) – that is, the ideas themselves – and this very process of serving such interests – reinforcing the power base of the status quo. A significant part of this is the process of 'stereotyping'.

An important distinction can be drawn between 'archetypes' and 'stereotypes'. An archetype is a 'typification' – that is, a set of typical characteristics and expectations we associate with a particular person, group or thing. It is a helpful way of simplifying the complexity of social reality and thus making sense of the world. It introduces and maintains a degree of stability and predictability. However, this helpful and constructive process can easily spill over into the much more harmful and destructive process of stereotyping. A stereotype is a fixed set of ideas that come as a 'package'. A set of characteristics is assumed to apply in total to a person or group that is stereotyped. For example, stereotypical ideas about older people include assumptions that they are deaf, inactive, dependent and incapable of making their own decisions. Not only are such assumptions patronizing, they are also very problematic, in so far as they distort reality by presenting oversimplified images of a complex reality.

What distinguishes an archetype from a stereotype is that we are likely to abandon an archetype as soon as we encounter information that negates our assumptions, whereas stereotypes tend to persist regardless of evidence or experience to the contrary. For example, someone who holds negative stereotypes about black people who meets a black person they get on with and feel positive towards, is likely to see that particular black person as an 'exception to the rule' and continue to hold negative views about black people in general, rather than abandon the stereotype.

This is a matter of assumptions. In forming a typification we make certain assumptions – often ideological assumptions – and, if we refuse to allow logic or evidence to challenge these, we run the risk of stereotyping, as we are more prepared to reject evidence than we are to reject our own ideology.

This concept of stereotyping is a particularly important one in relation to discrimination and oppression. Dominance, inequality and injustice are often maintained by means of stereotypes – for example of disabled people, gay men, lesbians or bisexuals. Stereotypes are therefore powerful tools of ideology, and are thus significant obstacles to the development of anti-discriminatory practice.

In terms of PCS analysis, ideology can be seen as the 'glue' that binds the levels together. It is ideology which acts as the vehicle of 'cultural transmission' between the **C** and **P** levels. Similarly, it is ideology which explains how the **C** level reflects, maintains and protects the **S** level by presenting social divisions as 'natural' and 'normal' and thus desirable. In short, the relationship between the levels is an ideological one, a reflection of the meeting point of the idea of power and the power of ideas.

Before leaving the topic of ideology, it is as well to point out that ideology is not an abstract force unconnected with human actions. Indeed, it is in, and through, human action that ideology comes into being. It is part of the complex interplay of individual and wider social forces, it is the bridge between the external objective world of social circumstances and the internal subjective world of meaning. As such, it is an existential concept, a dimension of human existence rather than an abstract form in its own right (Thompson, 1992).

The role of language

As ideology involves the communication of ideas, language is a central part of this process. It is therefore important to develop an understanding of the role of language in constructing and maintaining discrimination and oppression. Language is a major subject in its own right, and so the discussion here is necessarily selective (see Thompson, 2011b for a detailed discussion of the significance of language). Von Mende and Houlihan (2007) make apt comment when they point out that:

> Language forms the core of communication, and communication of socialization. It is through these that we expressively manifest who we are

to the outside world, and so they become vital for how we relate to others and how others perceive us.

(Von Mende and Houlihan, 2007, p. 217)

I shall focus on just two aspects, first, the discriminatory nature of some language forms, and second, a clarification of the terminology used in constructing a basis for anti-discriminatory practice.

Many words and expressions have derogatory, or overtly insulting overtones, while others are more subtle and less obvious in producing a discriminatory effect. For example, in the early days of concern about discrimination and language, the British Sociological Association (BSA) produced a set of guidelines on anti-sexist language which stated: 'When reference to both sexes is intended, a large number of phrases use the word "man" or other masculine equivalents (e.g. "father") and a large number of nouns use the suffix "man", thereby excluding women from the picture we present of the world.' Thus the use of 'masculine' language to refer to both men and women contributes to the 'invisibility' of women and thereby facilitates the persistence of the gender imbalance in terms of status and power. This is 'exclusive' language, as it has the effect of excluding women.

Similarly, the BSA produced a set of guidelines on anti-racist language, indicating which terms are appropriate and which are likely to have racist overtones. However, it is acknowledged that tackling these issues is difficult and far from straightforward:

> The issues are not always clear cut. There is disagreement as to whether some terms are acceptable or not and different political positions are aligned with different terms. Consequently, this guidance can only aim to promote an awareness of the issues in many instances rather than to prescribe or reinforce the use of particular terms.

The debate over terminology and racial discrimination will no doubt continue, and it is likely that a definitive lexicon of antiracism will remain elusive. Indeed, it is not simply a matter of distinguishing between 'taboo' words and 'OK' words, as in the sense of 'political correctness'. What is needed is not a simple list of proscribed words but, rather, an awareness of, and sensitivity to, the oppressive and discriminatory potential of language. This must be a fundamental part of anti-discriminatory practice, as the tendency to oversimplify language issues stands in the way of recognizing, and dealing with, the complexities of the power of language and their role in perpetuating patterns of discrimination and oppression. What we have to recognize is that choices always have consequences, and this applies just as much to our choice of language forms. To avoid our language use being discriminatory we therefore need to consider whether the language forms we use have positive, empowering consequences or negative, discriminatory ones.

Language is also a key aspect of ageism. As I have argued previously:

> Terms such as 'the elderly', 'the old', 'EMI' are commonly used but are, none the less, very dehumanizing – they 'depersonalize' the people to whom they refer; language can also patronize older people through the use of terms such as 'old dear', or by using first names without checking that this is acceptable. ... Language therefore plays a pivotal role with regard to dignity – it can either enhance it or act as a barrier to its realization.
>
> (Thompson, 1995a, pp. 11–12)

This passage is a good example of how the **C** level (culture as embodied in language) has a significant impact on the **P** level of our day-to-day practice. Furthermore, as Hugman (1994) has pointed out, referring to the work of Featherstone and Hepworth (1990): 'the language which surrounds old age and older people tends not to provide the materials with which to construct a positive identity' (p. 78).

Voice of experience 2.2

It was only when I started specializing in working with older people that I realized just how common ageist language was. You don't have to go very far before you come across an example of older people being described or spoken to in ways that reinforce ageist stereotypes. *Ayshea, a social worker in an older people team*

Much the same can be said of the language of disability. While depersonalized terms such as 'the elderly' are frowned upon by the anti-discriminatory movement, so too is the term 'the disabled'. A more appropriate term is 'disabled people' or 'people with disabilities' (see Chapter 6). But it is important that people understand why certain terms are problematic and best avoided, rather than just not use them because it is deemed 'not PC' to do so.

Language therefore needs to be used sensitively and critically in order to avoid negative connotations. Davis (1988) points out that even officially defined terms can be discriminatory. For example, he

distinguishes between the World Health Organization (WHO, 1980) definitions of impairment and disability (with their individualistic emphasis)
and those of the Union of the Physically Impaired Against Segregation
(UPIAS) which underline the social nature of disability – the restrictions
caused by social organization, rather than the impairment itself (UPIAS,
1976). This will be an important aspect of the discussions in Chapter 6.

Language therefore plays a significant part in the construction and
maintenance of discriminatory and oppressive forms of practice. However, it has often been argued that the use of language is secondary to the
good intentions of those using these terms. The argument goes: 'If people
use such terms in good faith without intending any ill-will towards
the groups concerned, surely it is petty to make an issue of the use of such
language?'

This seems a reasonable argument on the surface but, when we look
at it more closely, the pitfalls become visible. The major point we need to
recognize is that language is not simply a reflection of oppression (and
thus an innocuous route if paved with good intentions, it could be
argued), but actually constructs such oppression. Foucault uses the term
'discourse' to refer to the way in which language and other forms of communication act as the vehicle of social processes (see Foucault, 1977,
1979). For example, medical discourse not only reflects the power of the
medical profession but actively contributes to constructing, re-enacting
and thus perpetuating such power.

Discriminatory language therefore both reflects the discriminatory
culture and social structure in which we live, and also contributes to the
continuance of such discrimination. Language is not a passive receptacle;
it is an active encounter with the social world (Mooney and Evans, 2015).
Freire draws a similar conclusion:

> Human existence cannot be silent, nor can it be nourished by false
> words, but only by true words, with which men transform the world.
> To exist, humanly, is to name the world, to change it. Once named,
> the world reappears to the namers as a problem and requires of them
> a new naming.
>
> (Freire, 1972, pp. 60–1)

Language is part of the social world; indeed, it is one of the bridges
between the personal and the social and, as such, it cannot be neutral.
The language we use either reinforces discrimination through constructing it as 'normal' or contributes, in some small way at least, to undermining the continuance of a discriminatory discourse.

Rojek, Peacock and Collins also stressed the importance of language and its discriminatory potential when they argued that: 'the language which social workers are trained to use in order to free clients very often has the effect of imprisoning them anew' (1988, p. 1; see also Parton and O'Byrne, 2000, for an important discussion of these issues). This further underlines the need for a sensitivity to language and a critical approach to the forms of communication we commonly use. Indeed, it is largely for this reason that I shall now move on to clarify some of the key terms used in current attempts to promote anti-discriminatory practice. This is not intended as a glossary and is far from comprehensive in its coverage. However, I hope it will lead to a clearer understanding of some of the central issues, and thus make it easier to get to grips with the complexities of this intricate and thorny subject.

Discrimination

Unfair or unequal treatment of individuals or groups based on an actual or perceived difference; prejudicial behaviour acting against the interests of those people who characteristically tend to belong to relatively powerless groups within the social structure (women, ethnic minorities, old or disabled people and members of the working class in general). Discrimination is therefore a matter of social formation as well as individual or group behaviour.

Oppression

Inhuman or degrading treatment of individuals or groups; hardship and injustice brought about by the dominance of one group over another; the negative and demeaning exercise of power. It often involves disregarding the rights of an individual or group and is thus a denial of citizenship. Oppression arises as a result of unfair discrimination – that is, the disadvantages experienced as a result of discrimination have oppressive consequences.

Anti-discriminatory practice

An approach to practice which seeks to reduce, undermine or eliminate discrimination and oppression, specifically in terms of challenging sexism,

- power relations; and
- ideological legitimation based on biology.

There are also a number of others which have not been discussed here. For example, the concept of 'hegemony' is applicable across the board. This refers to the ideological dominance of one group over another or over a range of groups. One group, or 'social collectivity' (for example, men, white people, able-bodied people) gain power, status, position, prestige or some other advantage at the expense of other, less socially favoured groups (women, black or disabled people) and continue to maintain such dominance through the power of ideas which reinforce the 'naturalness' of the status quo.

Hegemony is therefore closely linked to the notion of exploitation, although not necessarily in any deliberate or intentional sense. It is also closely linked with ideology, for it is primarily through the vehicle of ideology that hegemony operates. Clarke and Cochrane explain the link between ideology and hegemony when they comment that ideologies:

> try to organize and mobilize elements of common-sense knowledge as part of their world view and in support of the social interests they represent. Thus, dominant social classes will refer to, and make connections with, aspects of common-sense knowledge that reflect and support existing patterns of inequality and which legitimate the economic or political power of these dominant groups. Counter-ideologies will want to build connections with those other elements of common-sense thought that object to or are sceptical about the existing social order. ... The aim is to ensure that there appears to be no alternative to the vision of society being presented that is capable of winning tacit or active support from people across a wide social spectrum. Gramsci used the term 'hegemonic' to describe a political project that achieved these ends.
>
> (Clarke and Cochrane, 1998, p. 33)

Key point 2.2

There are different forms of discrimination and different aspects, but we must not lose sight of the fact these 'dimensions of experience' are parts of a meaningful whole for the people concerned. They should not be seen in isolation.

Part of the ideological basis of hegemony is the idea of an 'out group', a group of people defined in negative terms and assigned an inferior status. This can be recognized as part of the process of discrimination and oppression and is thus a further commonality.

It is important that social workers are aware of the common threads and are able to respond to them accordingly – through resisting or weakening their influence and softening or preventing their impact. The commonalities are also an important part of avoiding the development of a divisive 'hierarchy of oppressions', as discussed in Chapter 1. Understanding the common themes is a major aspect of fighting the common enemies, those of discrimination and oppression. However, there are also significant differences between the multiple forms of oppression. It would be a mistake, both analytically and tactically, to concentrate exclusively on the commonalities without paying due heed to the important differences.

Practice focus 2.3

Darren had worked in a day centre for disabled people where he took a keen interest in issues of rights and equality. When he moved to a centre for older people, he expected to be able to continue his work on empowerment and was looking forward to challenging ageism in much the same way as he had tackled disablism in his previous job. However, he was soon to be disappointed as he found that many of the older people showed little or no interest in rights issues. At first, Darren was very worried by this as he felt that he would not be able to achieve any progress in his new job. However, after a little while, he regained his confidence and came to the conclusion that empowerment was not impossible, but he would have to make adjustments. His experience of dealing with one form of oppression could not be imported wholesale and uncritically into working with people experiencing another form of oppression.

It is beyond the scope of this book to give a detailed and thorough exposition of the differences, and so I shall restrict myself to a small selection by way of illustration of the wider field. Race and gender issues can be contrasted with age issues in at least two ways:

1 In the former cases, there is wide public awareness of the problems of discrimination and considerable sympathy in some quarters for supporting anti-discrimination measures. However, there is a much lower level of public awareness of ageism, and so ageist behaviours, assumptions and comments are much less likely to be challenged.

2 The people affected by discrimination on the grounds of age (or disability) are subject to the dangers of 'medicalization' (Powell, 2006). That is, old or disabled people are construed as 'ill' (and thus 'invalidated' – Laing, 1967; Laing and Cooper, 1971) in a way which women and black people are generally not.

There are also varying levels of publicity given to the areas and different levels of public awareness of the issues, both within social work in particular and within the wider community at large. As an example of this within social work, I have met many social workers who have told me the anti-discriminatory focus of their social work degree was almost exclusively on racism and sexism, with other forms of discrimination playing only a marginal role.

There are also differences in the ways in which racism and sexism are experienced and combated. For example, womanhood is not a totally homogeneous, undifferentiated entity (it intersects with class, race/ethnicity, age and so on). However, it is a much more homogeneous concept than that of race. There is, for example, no consensus as to which groups should be classified as 'black' – or 'Black' with a capital 'B' to emphasize that it is a political, rather than descriptive term (Williams, 1989, p. ix). The BSA guidelines on anti-racist language note, for example, that: 'some Asians in Britain object to the use of the word "black" being applied to them and some would argue that it also confuses a number of ethnic groups which should be treated separately'. There is a danger, however, of overemphasizing the differences and we should be clear about the need to focus on the commonalities and thus the common steps that can be taken to challenge discrimination and reduce or eliminate oppression.

There is a danger in placing too much emphasis on the disparate elements of oppression and thus failing to see the links between, for example, racism and sexism (Hill Collins, 2011) sexism and ageism (Arber, Davidson and Ginn, 2003) and so on. We can fail to see the patterns and common threads and thereby miss an opportunity for moving forward together as part of a wider anti-discrimination movement. It should also be remembered that the various oppressions are separated out for purposes of analysis and clarity of exposition, but are, in fact, dimensions of the same existence. People do not feel oppressions in isolation but, rather, as different but related aspects of what Sartre called 'lived experience' ('le vécu', Sartre, 1976).

This is a point which is particularly worthy of note in relation to the following chapters where the focus of attention falls on a particular form of oppression (beginning in Chapter 3, with sexism). The point again needs to be made that sexism, racism, ageism, disablism and so on are analytical categories and thus part of a wider and deeper social process (that of hegemony, social division and exploitation) rather than distinct and unrelated forms of discrimination.

Although substantially different, quantitatively and qualitatively, and in both a historical and contemporary sense, these forms of oppression share enough in common to justify a unified theoretical approach to tackle the relevant issues in each of these areas.

This chapter has contributed towards the task of establishing such a theory base. However, it would be naïve in the extreme to assume that the theoretical tools given here are sufficient for the task of developing a genuinely anti-discriminatory practice. This chapter, and indeed this book as a whole, can be only a beginning, a few relatively small, but none the less important steps in the right direction.

Food for thought

- Can you identify aspects of the culture you were brought up in that have discriminatory connotations (for example, in relation to gender roles)? How might these affect the way you practise as a social worker?

- Where would you locate yourself in the terms of the structure of society (class and race/ethnicity, for example)? How might your 'social location' affect your view of society in general and social work in particular?

- Can you identify ways in which the structure of society might affect clients, their circumstances and their problems? In what ways might you take these structural factors into consideration in your practice?

Further resources

Social divisions are a major feature of the sociological literature, and so a great deal has been written about them. For an introductory overview, see Payne (*Social Divisions*, 2006). Class in particular has a large literature base. A good starting point is Roberts (*Class in Contemporary Britain*, 2011). Lansley and Mack (*Breadline Britain: The Rise of Mass Poverty*, 2015) is an important text in relation to class inequalities.

PCS analysis is discussed at a more advanced level in *Promoting Equality* (Thompson, 2011a). Its applicability in making sense of power and empowerment is explored in Thompson (2007).

Bevan ('Poverty and Deprivation', 2002) provides a worked example of PCS analysis in relation to loss and grief issues.

Diversity is discussed briefly in Thompson (*Promoting Equality*, 2011a) and more fully in what has come to be seen as a classic work, Kandola and Fullerton (*Diversity in Action: Managing the Mosaic*, 1998) – see also Pincus (*Understanding Diversity: An Introduction to Class, Race, Gender, and Sexual Orientation*, 2011). The importance of language in social work is explored in Parton and O'Byrne (*Constructive Social Work: Towards a New Practice*, 2000). Thompson (*Effective Communication: A Guide for the People Professions*, 2011b) is devoted to an extensive discussion of communication and language and makes frequent reference to issues of discrimination and oppression. In particular, it warns of the dangers of oversimplifying these issues. Mooney and Evans (*Language, Society and Power*, 2015) provides a useful overview of the social and political implications of language.

An interesting discussion of stereotyping is to be found in Pickering (*Stereotyping: The Politics of Representation*, 2001).

Ideology and hegemony are discussed at an introductory level in Barker (*Cultural Studies*, 2008). *Promoting Equality* (2011a) also contains discussion of these topics.

Other important texts include: Dorling (*Inequality and the 1%*, 2014); Dorling (*Injustice: Why Social Inequality Still Persists*, 2015); Jones (*The Establishment and How They Get Away with It*, 2015); Stiglitz (*The Price of Inequality*, 2013); and Witcher (*Inclusive Equality: A Vision for Social Justice*, 2015).

CHAPTER 3

GENDER AND SEXISM

CHAPTER OVERVIEW

In this chapter you will:

- Appreciate the significance of gender as a key factor in people's lives and an important influence on how we experience our lives
- Learn about the ways in which sexism can be a major feature of the problems many people encounter, either a problem in its own right or something that makes other problems significantly worse
- Explore the implications of these issues for professional practice

Introduction

Gender is a fundamental dimension of human experience, revealing an ever-present set of differences between men and women. As de Beauvoir puts it in her classic text:

> In truth, to go for a walk with one's eye open is enough to demonstrate that humanity is divided into two classes of individuals whose clothes, faces, bodies, smiles, gaits, interests and occupations are manifestly different. Perhaps these differences are superficial, perhaps they are destined to disappear. What is certain is that they do most obviously exist.
>
> (de Beauvoir, 1972, pp. 14–15)

But it is not simply a matter of difference, of interesting and benign diversity. Abercrombie et al. argue that issues of gender (and gender inequality) now occupy a central place in sociological discussion:

> Gender is the social aspect of the differentiation of the sexes. Sociological discussion in this area recognizes that social rather than biological processes are the key to understanding the position of women (and of men) in society. Notions that a woman's biology, such as her capacity to bear children, determined the shape of her life have been replaced by

58

complex debates as to how different social processes interact to produce a great variety of patterns of gender relations. Emphasis has shifted towards understanding the diversity of the social practices which constitute gender in different nations, classes and generations.

> (Abercrombie et al., 2000, p. 193)

This notion of 'not just different but unequal' introduces the concept of sexism: inequality, discrimination and oppression on the grounds of gender – in short, male dominance or 'hegemony'. But what exactly is sexism? What are its constituent parts and what impact does it have on social work? These are important questions and open up a number of significant issues which can be seen as central to the theory and practice of social work. It is therefore important to clarify the basis and dimensions of sexism and it is with this task that we begin.

What is sexism?

Bullock and Trombley offer a useful definition of sexism:

> A word coined on the analogy of racism ... for a deep-rooted, often unconscious system of beliefs, attitudes, behaviour and institutions in which distinctions between people's intrinsic human worth are made on the grounds of their biological sex and gender roles.
>
> (Bullock and Trombley, 2000, p. 788)

The reference to 'beliefs, attitudes, behaviour and institutions' indicates that sexism operates at all three levels: **P**, **C** and **S**. The beliefs and actions of individuals, the cultural values and norms and the institutional or structural patterns all tend to display an inherent bias against women, producing a situation in which women:

- earn less than men and are more vulnerable to unemployment;
- tend to be concentrated in less prestigious and less secure forms of employment;
- do considerably more housework than men; and
- experience substantial inequalities in relation to housing, welfare benefits and health (see Abercrombie et al., 2000).

Sexism is closely linked to the concept of patriarchy, literally 'the law of the father'. Weber (1947) used this concept to refer to the dominance of men within the family. Its use, however, has been extended to refer to the dominance of men in general, as reflected in the distribution of power in society. In a classic feminist work Millett captured this point well when she argued that: 'the military, industry, technology, universities, science, political office, and finance – in short, every avenue of power within the society, including the coercive force of the police, is entirely in male hands' (1971, p. 25). Perhaps 'entirely' is an overstatement, but it none the less remains the case that power at a structural level is predominantly a male phenomenon.

Voice of experience 3.1

We did a project at university about gender inequalities. I already knew that it's a man's world in a lot of ways, but that project really hammered home for me just how many ways there are for sexism to make a worrying difference. *Marie, a social work student*

Sexism is therefore a set of beliefs, practices and institutional structures which reinforces, and is reinforced by, patriarchy. The two concepts are mutually supportive. In particular, patriarchal ideology promotes the traditional model of the family, (with the male breadwinner as provider, head of the household and defender of his territory, the wife and mother as nurturer and carer and their dependent children, whom they socialize into following in the footsteps of the appropriate role model – boys to grow up like daddy, girls to grow up like mummy.)

In fact, the links between patriarchy and the nuclear family are so great that the term 'familial ideology' has been coined to refer to the ideas base which seeks to legitimate these social relations. It reflects the view that the nuclear family, with clearly defined traditional gender roles is the right and natural way for people to live. This then becomes a two-way process. Familial ideology not only reflects traditional gender roles, but also creates the context in which such roles can be learned by children as they are brought up within the nuclear family.

The emphasis on the nuclear family as 'normal' thus defines other family forms as 'deviant' and undesirable. The pressure to conform to sex-appropriate roles within the patriarchal family is both a major part of the socialization process and a significant aspect of sexism. As Cohen and MacCartney argue:

> *families contain and reproduce inequalities*, both personally intimate and economically pivotal. For example, the division of labor and resources

within families usually privileges men, with women dominating unpaid housework and child-care while men hold privileged positions in the paid labor market.

(Cohen and MacCartney, 2007, p. 181)

An important constituent part of sexism, as referred to here is that of the sexual division of labour. Work tasks, both within and outside the home, tend to follow a gender-specific pattern. Women tend to be involved primarily in the domestic sphere of housework and childcare, while men are more closely associated with the public sphere of paid work and political life (Lister, 2003). The allocation of pay, status, leisure time and other rewards shows a distinct bias in favour of men at the expense of women.

Rowbotham (1973) was among the first to link this to capitalism and the marxist notion of men as producers (that is, workers producing material wealth) and women as reproducers (that is, childbearers and nurturers of the workforce). However, Pascall (1997), while recognizing the contribution of this marxist analysis to social policy, bemoans the overemphasis on production and thus relative neglect of reproduction. She therefore argues for a greater understanding of the role of the family in the sexual division of labour. In particular, there is a need for greater attention to be paid to the ways in which social policy (including – potentially – forms of social work practice that uncritically accept traditional gender roles) reinforces familial ideology and the sexism inherent within it. Pascall comments:

Support for the breadwinner/dependant form of family has entrenched the dependency of women in marriage as well as the difficulties of living outside such families, of forming different kinds of relationships, and of leaving particular unhappy marriages.

(Pascall, 1997, p. 25)

This is an important point and will be relevant to the discussions below of the interrelationships between social policy, social work and sexism/patriarchy.

Practice focus 3.1

Frank was an experienced social worker who specialized in family work. He took great pride in his work and tried very hard to make sure that he did a good job. He was therefore very disconcerted when one of the families he worked with made a complaint against him. A single mother had complained about his 'old-fashioned' attitude towards women and his apparent disapproval of single-parent

▶

families without a traditional 'breadwinner'. This came as a complete surprise to Frank and forced him to rethink his views about women and families and the assumptions he had been making.

A further aspect of sexism relates specifically to sexuality and the implicit (or sometimes explicit) assumption that male sexuality is a strong and 'difficult to resist' force. This assumption is then often used, in part at least, to justify or excuse male aggression against women. Weeks (1986) refers to this as the 'Biological Imperative' and it is yet another example of a biological argument being used as a basis for legitimating social relations, power and dominance. Weeks comments:

> The idea that there are differences between peoples is not in itself dangerous. What is peculiar about sexuality is that certain differences have been seen as so fundamental that they become divisions and even antagonisms. At best, there is the argument, that though men and women may be different, they can still be equal. At worst, assumptions about the forceful nature of the sexual drive have been used to legitimize male domination over women.
>
> (Weeks, 1986, p. 47)

This 'dominance' can be seen to go a step further and emerge as sexual violence. The seriousness of violence against women is something that has not yet been fully appreciated in social work (Harne and Radford, 2008; Radford, 2001). For a variety of reasons, including the at times less than helpful response of the law enforcement agencies, a major proportion of these incidents go unreported and do not therefore appear in the crime statistics.

These issues are also relevant to our understanding of, and response to, child sexual abuse, as will become clear in the next section concerning the implications of sexism.

Key point 3.1

Men and women are different in many ways, but such difference does not justify the unfairness involved in sexism. If we are not tuned in to the significance of gender-related discrimination, we run the risk of reinforcing and exacerbating the unfairness involved.

Patriarchy, then, is one of the *structural* dimensions of society which is strongly associated with the sexist *culture* which demeans and disempowers women and thus sows the seeds for the cultivation of *personal* prejudice in terms of both attitudes and behaviour. The taken-for-granted nature of sexism at an individual level thereby promotes and protects the patriarchal structure. Thus, sexist ideology keeps the wheels of oppression turning.

But what impact does this have on social work? In what ways does social work fit into this picture? It is these issues I shall now address.

The implications for social work

One of the major implications for social work is the need to rethink radically the male-dominated and masculine-orientated basis of traditional social work theory. As Mullender comments:

> It is not possible to understand the personal or social world without taking a gendered perspective. We cannot intervene appropriately in people's lives unless we see how women remain disadvantaged in contemporary society, and how both men and women are expected to play over-rigid and falsely dichotomized roles and relationship expectations.
>
> (Mullender, 2008, p. 313)

Sexism raises many issues for social workers seeking to develop anti-discriminatory practice. While this text cannot address all of them, we can at least begin to explore some of them.

It has long been recognized that social work operates at the boundaries of 'normality' and 'deviance' (see, for example, Pearson, 1975) and so it is important that we recognize that our conceptions of normality are 'gendered'. That is, we need to become sensitive to the gender issues involved in the notion of 'normal'. For example, the concept of a 'normal' family, as commonly used, is likely to be a patriarchal family; 'normal' child-rearing practices are also gender specific – when we speak of 'good-enough parenting', we are, more often than not, talking of 'good enough mothering', father remaining relatively invisible.

It is therefore an easy step from taking 'normality' for granted to reinforcing stereotypical expectations of men and women. Carlen and Worrall comment on the expectations of a 'normal' woman:

> Being a normal woman means coping, caring, nurturing and sacrificing self-interest to the needs of others. It also means being intuitively sensitive

to those needs without them being actively spelt out. It means being *more than man*, in order to support and embrace Man. On the other hand, femininity is characterized by lack of control and dependence. Being a normal woman means needing protection ... It means being childlike, incapable, fragile and capricious. It is being *less than man* in order to serve and defer to Man.

(Carlen and Worrall, 1987, p. 3)

A clear implication for social workers, therefore, is the need to develop a *critical* approach which questions and challenges everyday assumptions and thereby gets underneath the ideological gloss of 'normality'.

The converse of this situation also applies. That is, not only can social work be seen to reinforce sexism if a critical approach is not adopted, but sexism can also be seen to be a major factor underpinning many of the problems social workers are asked to tackle. The discrimination and oppression inherent in sexism are, of course, not without cost to the women concerned.

Poverty is one example of this, as women have more restricted access to resources than men. This produces a situation which has come to be known as the 'feminization of poverty' (Spicker, 2001), as so many women are reliant upon either men or state benefits for financial support (Zartler, 2002). A related concept is that of 'secondary poverty', the fact that women (and children), even in relatively financially secure households, are often starved of resources – the man of the household taking a disproportionate amount of the family income to follow his leisure interests or other pursuits (Bryson, 1999). Similarly, Lister's (2004) important work on poverty recognizes that it is generally women (and children) who bear the main brunt of poverty.

The links between poverty and the problems social work clients experience have been clearly established and are well documented (Bateman, 2008). The fact that women constitute the majority of social work clients adds weight to the 'feminization of poverty' thesis and also underlines the linkages between gender, oppression and social work.

Poverty has also been associated with mental health problems and with depression in particular. Depression is also significant in terms of gender: women are heavily over-represented as far as this disorder is concerned (Appignanesi, 2008; Fawcett and Karban, 2005). This is relevant for social workers at two levels:

1 Specifically in terms of mental health social work and the significance of gender for this type of work.

2   More generally in relation to a range of social work situations in which depression plays a part: childcare (including child protection); loss and grief; work with older people and so on.

Brown and Harris (1978) undertook what has come to be recognized as a classic study of the incidence of depression in women and sought to uncover the underlying factors. They were surprised by the relatively high frequency of depression among women, especially in urban areas. A number of 'vulnerability factors' were identified (for example, a low level of intimacy with one's partner) and these, in turn, tend to lead to low self-esteem. The low self-esteem of many women therefore leaves them much more prone to depression.

But Brown and Harris emphasized that these are sociological factors, to do with the position of women in society, rather than purely psychological matters. They comment that depression is not only relatively common but also:

> fundamentally related to social values since it arises in a context of hopelessness consequent upon the loss of important sources of reward or positive value. A woman's own social milieu and the broader social structure are critical because they influence the way in which she thinks about the world and thus the extent of this hopelessness; they determine what is valued, as well as what is lost and how often, and what resources she has to face the loss.
>
> (Brown and Harris, 1978, p. 270)

Although Brown and Harris did not refer specifically to sexism, it is clear that the same issues are applicable. Indeed, PCS analysis is highly compatible with their work – the psychological level being embedded within the wider cultural milieu and social structure.

Reference was made above to child protection work, and once again gender issues can be seen to be relevant here too. It has long been recognized that the concept of 'dangerous *families*' in reality relates to 'dangerous *mothers*' (Parton and Parton, 1989). Mothers are seen to have primary responsibility for children (this is a key part of patriarchal ideology) and are therefore held responsible when things go wrong. Even when the mother herself is not the abuser, she is often deemed to be culpable by virtue of the fact that she has failed to protect the child. Parenting is seen primarily as mothering. Poor parenting, neglect or abuse are therefore construed mainly as a failure on the part of women.

Despite the fact that the majority of sexual abuse cases involve male perpetrators, the focus remains on the role of the mother. It is her role to protect the child in general and this includes protection from the powerful and driven male sexuality to which Weeks referred in the quotation above. Implicit blame therefore tends to be attributed to the female's 'failure to protect', rather than the male's proclivity to abuse. Saraga captured these points well in the following passage:

> If abuse is seen as something wrong in the family, then decisions about 'protection' of the child focus on whether or not the family is or can be helped to become a safe place, or whether the child should be removed from home. In practice, much of the discussion focuses on the mother's role, in particular asking whether she 'knew' about the abuse, whether she 'colluded' and whether she 'failed to protect' her child. By conveying a meaning that she *should* have known, the intervention may serve to strengthen her denial. In contrast, a practice influenced by a feminist perspective emphasizes the responsibility of the individual abuser, and therefore aims to remove him rather than the child from the home, so that the child can remain in the non-abusing part of the family. It also recognizes that the mother has herself suffered a loss and betrayal, that she may need help in her own right to accept what has happened in order to be able to make decisions, and to support her child.
>
> (Saraga, 1993, p. 77)

The prevalence of the viewpoint Saraga is rejecting here is a clear example of the strength and depth of the influence of patriarchal ideology. Women are cast as primary carers and so, in situations of child abuse, they find themselves in a 'no-win' situation. If they are the abusers (and we shall come on to discuss this below), they have failed as mothers and thus failed as people. Where it is the menfolk who are the abusers, the women have failed in their duty to protect (and, in the eyes of some, also failed to 'keep their man happy'). Men, by contrast, tend not to be charged with a failure to protect and, even where they are the perpetrator, some allowance is often made for their behaviour, based on essentialist notions of male aggression and unrestrained sexuality being 'natural' (the 'Biological Imperative').

Physical abuse of children has often been described as an abuse of parental power, or the power of adults over children in general. In sexual abuse, the gender dimension is more apparent, as the choice of a child as a sexual partner can be seen as an example of male sexuality as a form of power (see, for example, Segal, 2007) and sexual abuse as an abuse of such power. Indeed, in 1989, Corby argued that it was only the efforts of feminists that had brought the problems of child sexual abuse to light and he referred to Rush (1981), who had contended that issues such as child sexual abuse and child pornography were not being tackled because men in power did not take them seriously.

Ong (1985) also made an important contribution to developing our knowledge base in discussing the concept of 'wonderful children' which refers to the tendency to idealize children and concentrate on the positive aspects of bringing them up. The pressures, stresses and pains are paid scant attention and tend to be 'swept under the carpet', thus placing immense additional pressure on women to conform to the idealized norm of a happy, contented mother. In reporting her study of mothers and children at a family centre, she comments:

> [Mothers] are often feeling guilty that they cannot perceive their children in positive ways, and fail to see that this is largely related to factors outside their personal power. Taking women's own experiences as a point of departure, investigating the limitations in their mothering context, can probably instigate more positive change than insisting that all children are wonderful.
>
> (Ong, 1985, p. 105)

The common ideological view of children as 'wonderful' is therefore an additional source of oppression for women.

Practice focus 3.2

Liz had been keen to become a mother, even though she was only 17. However, she had not thought through the consequences and was not prepared for what it would entail. Her boyfriend, Steve, was horrified to find she was pregnant and very quickly disappeared from the scene. Liz's parents were very annoyed with her and offered her only very limited support. Within six months of giving birth, Liz felt under immense pressure with the very limited support and she became increasingly withdrawn and uncommunicative. The health visitor was sufficiently concerned to make a referral to Social Services.

A further implication of sexism for social work is the casting of women in a caring role. The idea that the community care of disabled, mentally disordered or elderly people is primarily care by the family – which, in turn, amounts to care by women – originates from the work of Finch and

Groves in 1983. However, Mullender shows that the issue of women as carers is still a very significant one for us to be aware of:

> Considerations of gender in community care began with a focus on women as carers which remains real, even today. Although there are also substantial numbers of male carers, they remain mainly husbands and mainly elderly. The person who gives up work, leisure or health to care for a dependant is far more likely to be a woman. Minority ethnic carers and gay and lesbian partners who care remain amongst the most neglected groups. The idea that informal carers should have attention paid to their needs is only slowly influencing practice.
>
> (Mullender, 2008, p. 314)

She goes on to make the important point that:

> Carers in residential care are almost all female. The assumption that this automatically makes them suitable for the work blocks access to training, support and promotion. Many black women carry a double burden of caring, acting as both low-paid care or nursing staff and as key family and community supports.
>
> (Mullender, 2008, p. 314)

There is therefore a clear need to avoid making the assumption that women's roles as carers are 'natural' or that men are not 'cut out' for caring (Thompson and Bates, 2002). As Fisher has argued, the assumption that men will find caring difficult:

> allows service providers to cite the carer's masculine gender as evidence of the need for service. It allows the myth of the incompetent man to be reproduced, and to be imposed on male carers and on care receivers.
>
> (Fisher, 1994, p. 673)

Patriarchal ideology is therefore very significant in relation to caring roles and something that we should be very wary of reinforcing.

This takes us back to the concept of familial ideology which can be seen to be implicit in social policy. While the family as a set of living arrangements has a number of advantages, we should not forget that:

1 Traditional family roles and the patriarchal assumptions on which they are based, can have a profoundly alienating effect on women by restricting life chances, imposing high and often unrealistic expectations in terms of undertaking caring duties and so on.

2 The family is a potentially very destructive institution and, given that women act as the lynchpin of the family in the domestic sphere, it is likely that they will suffer the greatest effects and, indeed, be allocated the greater share of the blame. This is particularly significant for social work, operating as it does, at the intersection of conflicting forces, within the family and the wider social sphere.

Social workers therefore need to adopt a critical stance towards the family, as the traditional social policy eulogy of the family conceals a large number of patriarchal assumptions which fuel the sexism which oppresses women by chaining them to the domestic sphere of caring and nurturing. But social work also needs to look at itself to see sexism as, for example, in the sexual division of labour to be found within social work organizations. Women form the majority of social work clients and social work staff, and yet they form a relatively small minority of senior managers (Coulshed et al. 2006).

Hayward (2005) argues that women managers face additional pressures, in so far as they have to operate within a predominantly masculine environment and ethos in which leadership skills can be seen as 'unfeminine'. She argues that, rather than trying to justify their place in the 'man's world' of management by adopting male tactics, women can make a positive contribution on their own terms:

> Are we finally realizing that the answer lies in using our own unique female skills rather than falling down as we've done in the past by trying to copy the boys, bearing the weight of an outdated and ill-fitting 'macho' image that we previously felt was the only way forward...?
>
> (Hayward, 2005, p. 1)

Social work agencies are very clearly not immune from the workings of patriarchy and, indeed, very much reflect them. Occupational segregation in social work is based on a 'sexual division of labour', with women occupying the majority of lower status, lower paid jobs while men occupy the majority of more highly paid, higher status posts (Coulshed, Mullender et al., 2006; Fröschl, 2002). This has major implications for attempts to develop anti-sexist practice. It needs to be recognized that such endeavours involve 'swimming against the tide' within a masculine-dominated organizational structure and ethos.

There are, of course, very many other implications for social work deriving from sexism, but space does not permit a more extensive exposition of the issues here. However, I hope the examples given here have raised awareness sufficiently for readers to pursue other issues through further reading and discussion.

The question of how we take forward anti-sexist practice is of course a major one and follows on from the discussion here. However, before tackling these issues, we need to be clear about the contribution of feminist theory to this area of social work. In short, it would be unwise to begin to address practice issues without first exploring the theory base – the theoretical formulations of a now well-established tradition of feminist thought. There is now a clear basis for the further development of anti-sexist practice as the emergence of a specifically feminist school of social work has shown (see White, 2006). It is therefore important to understand at least the basics of feminist theory.

Voice of experience 3.2

I really enjoyed the family therapy course I did and we had some really interesting discussions about how gender works in families in such complex and fascinating ways. It really brought home to me how much attention I need to pay to gender issues in families if I am not going to add to the existing problems.
Karen, a children and families social worker

The feminist response

Williams (1989) has helpfully presented an account of six different forms of feminism and draws out some of the similarities and differences. This indicates that there is no one consistent and uniform feminism, no simple consensus on the factors underlying male domination and the strategies required to tackle these.

However, this is not to say that there are no common themes or points of agreement. Indeed, they all share a focus on the critique of patriarchy and the need to establish a fairer society in which women are no longer marginalized, alienated and pushed into secondary roles. They also share the belief that 'the personal is political'. This has several levels of meaning:

1 The domestic private sphere also contributes to the wider public and political sphere. For example, housework and childcare are not marginal to the economy but do, in fact, play a key role in maintaining the workings of economic structures and processes.

2   The personal sphere is one dominated by issues of power. Power is not simply a matter of macro structures relating to large-scale social issues; it also revolves around personal relationships, identity and other such microstructural aspects of social life.

3   The family is the locus of political struggle. Power, conflict and domination are common aspects of family life. In particular, the power of men over women manifests itself most clearly in the family home in terms of the sexual division of labour, the allocation of leisure time and so on.

4   Gender is socially constructed (that is, it hinges on the social significance attached to the differences between men and women), rather than biologically determined. Gender therefore has wider social and political connotations.

5   The oppression of women, and the problems they experience arising from this, are not only 'private troubles' but also 'public issues' (Mills, 1970).

6   Personal problems have their roots in political structures and political structures are reinforced by a particular form of personal relations (patriarchy).

Feminism therefore seeks to:

1   *Politicize the personal*: to draw attention to the political nature and basis of the alienation and oppression of women; and

2   *Personalize the political*: to engage women in the collective political struggle for equality and equal rights.

The latter is, of course, premised on the heightened awareness achieved by the former. How this struggle should be taken forward is the subject of fierce debate and will no doubt continue to be for some time yet.

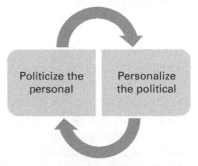

Figure 3.1 Politicize the personal; personalize the political

The early form of feminism has been labelled 'liberal feminism' and its basic tenets continue to be adhered to by a number of theorists and activists. The emphasis in liberalism is on the individual. Individuals are expected to attain differing levels of achievement within social life and the marketplace. This is felt to be natural and desirable provided that no individual or group of individuals is unfairly disadvantaged. And this is where liberal feminism comes in – women are felt to be handicapped in competing for jobs, status, power and so on as a result of sexism.

Liberal feminism therefore sees the way forward as a combination of campaigning for equal opportunities generally, educating people about the problems of discrimination, and in general allowing a fairer basis on which women can compete, on an individual basis, with men. Change is seen as gradual, incremental and based on specific targets for reform.

The liberal feminist focus is, in terms of PCS analysis, very much at the **P** level, the personal or individual. And it is this which has been the major source of criticism of this approach. The individualism inherent in liberal feminism is castigated for failing to take account of the wider aspects, particularly the structural nature of power relations and the institutional, rather than personal, sources of discrimination and oppression. It is seen as rather a naïve approach which tinkers with superficial aspects of the problem, rather than tackling the social and political roots. This is sometimes expressed in comical (but none the less serious) terms as 'rearranging the deckchairs on the Titanic' – that is, maintaining a blinkered view of a structurally based problem.

However, we should not dismiss liberal feminism altogether. It is more helpful to see it as not going far enough, rather than going in the wrong direction. The need, therefore, is not to reject liberal feminism, but rather to transcend it. Indeed, liberal feminists could argue that they have achieved significant steps forward in terms of anti-discrimination legislation and a higher level of awareness of gender inequality, while more structurally based approaches have achieved little or nothing. This is an important argument for anti-sexist social work and one to which I shall return below.

An alternative perspective is that of radical feminism. By contrast with liberalism, radical feminism focuses on underlying structural and power issues which are seen to hinge on the key concept of *patriarchy*. In radical feminism the dominance of men is seen as a historical constant, a ubiquitous feature of male-dominated relations. Regardless of the type of society – capitalist, pre-capitalist, communist or whatever – men are everywhere to be found in positions of power, including central and local government, economic institutions, the judiciary, the professions and so on.

As we have noted, ideology (in this case, patriarchal ideology) operates on the basis of assumed natural or biological bases of women's roles in society. Drawing on this idea, radical feminism emphasizes the part played by repro- duction and the family structures and ideology that have been constructed around the notion of women as primarily mother figures, thus allowing men to take up the powerful father role (hence the word patriarchy).

The strength of the radical perspective is that it recognizes the struc- tural dimension of women's oppression and therefore goes much further than the liberal approach which would leave existing power structures relatively untouched. Radical feminism, as the name implies, identifies the need to tackle the problems at the root, to redress the power balance between men and women, and this cannot be done by piecemeal reform alone. A more comprehensive programme of social change is called for.

The weakness of this approach is its ahistorical nature. It sees the domi- nance of men as universal – both across cultures and through history. Thus it has been criticized for placing too much emphasis on the biologi- cal underpinnings of sexism and not enough on historical, sociopolitical factors. Marxist-feminism – or socialist feminism as it is often called – shares radical feminism's emphasis on the structural and power base of the oppression of women. However, unlike the radical approach marxist- feminism focuses not on the biological roots of sexism, but rather on its historical and political roots.

Marxist-feminism sees patriarchy as a structure which supports and reinforces capitalism. The family is seen as a microcosm of wider society in which women represent the proletariat (the exploited class) and men the bourgeoisie (the exploiters) (Engels, 1976/1844). A central part of this is the sexual division of labour, as discussed earlier in this chapter. Men are socialized into the role of workers in the public sphere – the producers – while women are socialized into the roles of wives and mothers in the pri- vate sphere – the reproducers. This arrangement is well suited to capitalism, as it produces a workforce which is 'serviced' from within the family. In addition, it provides a 'reserve army of labour', a secondary (female) work- force which can be recruited when the economy expands or in exceptional circumstances (for example, men going off to war) and dispensed with when they are no longer required. This is facilitated by the fact that women tend to be located lower down the occupational hierarchy.

Marxist-feminism recognizes the dual oppressions of capitalism (related to class) and patriarchy (related to gender) and the interrelationship between the two. As Williams has so succinctly put it: 'there can be no socialism without women's liberation, and no women's liberation without socialism' (1989, p. 57). The marxist version of feminism seeks to locate patriarchy within the context of a materialist analysis. That is, patriarchy is not simply a reflection of biological differences between men and women. Rather, it is closely related to the production of material life – that is, the economic base.

This link with the economy is precisely one of the strong points of marxist-feminism. It succeeds in relating the power of men over women to that of the capitalist class over the working class.

This emphasis on class is perhaps also its main weakness. The main focus of explanation is the economic base and the class divisions on which it rests. This leads to a relative weakness in terms of explaining the dominance of men over women in non-capitalist societies, for example, agrarian societies.

In recent years a further approach to feminism has become more firmly established, namely postmodernist feminism. This approach follows post-modernist thought in challenging the notion of fixed identities. It argues the case for seeing gender identities as socially constructed, rather than biologically fixed – see Ives (2007) for further discussion.

There are, of course, other forms of feminism which have something to offer to an understanding of women's oppression. But what is clear is that there is no one right answer, no definitive feminist school of thought. The debates and struggles continue and, from a social work point of view, the positive thing to note is that the issues are now more firmly established on the professional agenda than ever before.

The approaches to feminism are not static and fixed. Literature on this subject continues to be published. And, what is perhaps most significant is that there is now a growing body of literature on feminism and social welfare – see the 'Further resources' section below.

Sexism and men

There are two aspects to the question of men and sexism: first, what impact does sexism have on men? And, second, what part can men play in undermining, reducing or eliminating sexism?

Key point 3.2

Sexism is a complex phenomenon that has a profound negative impact on women and, in some ways, on men too. We therefore have to recognize that it is important for women and men to support one another in tackling the discrimination and oppression involved.

While the actions and attitudes of men are often a significant source of pressure and difficulty for women as a result of the potent and far-reaching influence of sexist ideology, it cannot be said that sexism is unproblematic for men. There are clearly many ways in which men do benefit from the power and privilege invested in them by patriarchy. However, it must also be recognized – and this is a very important potential source of change – that men also suffer as a result of sexism (although clearly not to the same extent or depth as women, see Thompson, 1995b). The negative impact of sexism on men can be seen to include the following elements:

● Certain emotions are regarded as feminine and thus 'off limits' to many men (Jansz, 2000).

● Many men die as a result of not seeking medical help in the early stages of a life-threatening illness (see Luck, Bamford and Williamson, 2000).

● Many people die or are injured as a result of ritualized displays of masculinity – high-speed car chases, for example. As Wilkinson puts it:

Although more unequal societies are more male-dominated and the position of women deteriorates relative to men, men's death rates are even more adversely affected by inequality than women's.

(Wilkinson, 2005, p. 215)

● Many men are drawn into a life of crime because, in part at least, they are misguidedly expressing their masculinity.

● Divorced fathers are far less likely to gain custody of their children.

● Men, like women, can feel alienated and disaffected as a result of culturally defined gender role expectations and the limitations they impose.

It is now increasingly being recognized that the dehumanization inherent in sexism as the basis presents an argument for men adopting a pro-feminist stance in opposing sexism (Segal, 2007; Thompson and Bates, 2002). This is to recognize that anti-sexism is a battle to be fought not only by women, but also by men, partly for their own emotional emancipation and partly for humanitarian reasons as a step towards the dissolution of oppressive structures and practices. It would be naïve indeed to assume that men would readily give up the advantages of patriarchy but this should not deter us from seeing the benefits of anti-sexism for both women and men. As Segal comments:

> Why feminism? Because its most radical goal, both personal and collective, has yet to be realized: a world which is a better place not just for some women, but for all women. In what I call a socialist feminist vision, that would be a far better world for boys and men, as well.
>
> (Segal, 1999, p. 232)

Men therefore have a part to play in furthering the cause of anti-sexism. A major aspect of this is the need to become sensitive to the part we play in reproducing sexist structures and cultural patterns in and by our actions and attitudes. In short, both men and women need to be aware of how their actions (the **P** level) can avoid falling into the trap of reinforcing and reproducing the sexism inherent in the **C** and **S** levels – and, indeed, can even go so far as challenging those patterns and structures. Mullender captures the point well when she argues that:

> In social work education and practice, men can usually come together in groups to work on the emotional barriers to the feminine in themselves – to feelings and vulnerabilities – which drive them towards aggressive competitiveness and, at the same time, keep women and gay men oppressed. Men need to consider how they can better support women colleagues – at every level from campaigning for crèches and sharing the care of dependants, to tackling sexual harassment and violence – and be part of a more appropriate service for women and children and a more confrontational practice with abusive or exploitative men.
>
> (Mullender, 2008, p. 316)

Practice focus 3.3

Adriana found working in a male-dominated team quite trying at times. She grew tired of some of the comments and sexist assumptions that were commonly made. She did not complain about this situation, however, until one particularly difficult day when she felt the need to express her anger. Some of the men in the team became very defensive but, to her great surprise and relief, two of her male colleagues were very supportive indeed and made strenuous efforts to rid the team of its sexist overtones and tendencies. She recognized that men too had a part to play in challenging sexism.

Towards anti-sexist practice

Although there is a growing body of literature on anti-sexist theory and policy, this is unlikely to have an impact unless it is put into practice. It is therefore necessary to focus on some of the ways in which anti-sexist practice can be made a reality. Of course, there can be no single 'formula' approach to putting anti-sexist theory into practice, but identifying some broad principles can I hope help us move in the right direction.

1 The aim of social work intervention is empowerment, not adjustment (Thompson, 2007). The social work task should not be to help women to adjust to their 'rightful' place in the family, but rather to assist them in gaining the power to overcome or challenge the oppression they experience. The personal is, after all, political.

2 An important, indeed major, part of this is the need to avoid stereo-typical assumptions. We should not assume, for example, that the male is the head of the household and the primary decision maker in a two-parent family. If we are not careful, assessing family dynamics can be reduced to jumping to sexist conclusions.

3 Similarly, in childcare cases, in addition to focusing on the child(ren), work should be directed towards parents rather than simply mothers. If not, we run the risk of 'mother blaming' and reinforcing the notion that women carry the primary responsibility for the family.

4 The sexist implications of the notion of 'community care' need to be addressed. This entails resisting the pressure to push women into caring roles. Sexist ideology leads us to believe that it is 'natural' for women to be carers and this can, unless we guard against it, allow us to ignore or marginalize the intense pressures which can be inherent in the caring role.

5 Familial ideology reinforces sexism by emphasizing the positives of family life and playing down the negatives. Social workers are likely to be well aware of the destructive capabilities of families, but may none the less be seduced by familial ideology into uncritically promoting the value of the family. Social work practice needs to be based on a balanced view of the family which recognizes both its strengths and its weaknesses.

6 Clients too are strongly influenced by familial ideology in particular and sexist ideology in general. While the primary task of social work is not

the dissolution of sexism, consciousness raising is often necessary to help service users understand how sexism may be contributing to their problems or acting as a barrier to the solution of their problems. This parallels the radical social work principle of helping people recognize the political basis of many of the problems commonly experienced (poverty, bad housing, alienation and so on).

7   The strengths perspective (Saleebey, 2006) has warned against the dangers of portraying clients in unduly negative terms as 'helpless' or 'not coping' in order to gain additional resources for them. This can be seen to apply especially to women, as this misguided tactic has the effect of producing enforced dependency and is therefore one to be avoided.

8   Women are 'invisible' within a male-dominated society in so far as their achievements and contributions are rarely given due credit. Social workers need to avoid this trap and appropriately value women, their thoughts, feelings and work. At a micro level social work can contribute to enhanced self-esteem for women clients (and staff) and at a macro level play at least a small part in the breaking down of the sexist devaluation of women.

9   Sexual harassment is also an important issue. Unwelcome sexual attention in its various forms can cause considerable distress to women and can lead to lower levels of confidence and job performance. This can apply to both women colleagues and clients. Although much sexual harassment is unintentional, based on an insensitivity to women's needs and feelings (and thus a reflection of cultural assumptions at the C level about women as sexual objects), it is none the less oppressive (Thompson, 2000b). Anti-sexist social work must challenge intentional forms of harassment and develop sufficient sensitivity to avoid unintentional forms.

10 Anti-sexist practice involves challenging dominant discriminatory attitudes, values, practices and structures. It entails 'problematizing' – that is, taking everyday, apparently unproblematic matters and showing just how problematic they can be, highlighting just how discriminatory and oppressive they really are. This includes Berger's (1966) notion of 'debunking' or Mills's (1970) 'sociological imagination'. In short, it amounts to questioning assumptions about men and women in society and involves adopting a critical approach.

There are many more points and examples which could be given to build on these basics. Indeed, it should be recognized that sexism is so pervasive and so deeply ingrained in society in general and social work in particular that we should develop as extensive a repertoire as possible of strategies for promoting anti-sexist practice.

Food for thought

- Consider your own gender. How might the way you have been brought up as a woman or a man influence your practice as a social worker?
- Can you identify any ways in which gender can be a key factor in the problems social workers attempt to deal with?
- The majority of policy makers and senior managers are men. What difference might this make to how social work services are delivered?
- Sexist stereotypes can be very damaging. Can you identify a number of common stereotypical assumptions about men and women? How might you avoid relying on such stereotypes?

Further resources

Mullender ('Engendering the Social Work Agenda', 2008) is a very good short introductory account. White (*The State of Feminist Social Work*, 2006) provides a very good analysis of a wide range of issues relating to gender and social work, as do Gruber and Stefanov (*Gender in Social Work: Promoting Equality*, 2002).

Coulshed et al. (*Management in Social Work*, 2006) address gender in relation to management in a social care context, while Wilson (2003) explores gender and organizational behaviour.

Arber, Davidson and Ginn (*Gender and Ageing: Changing Roles and Relationships*, 2003) provide a very illuminating account of women, and old age, while Appignanesi (*Mad, Bad and Sad: A History of Women and the Mind Doctors from 1800 to the Present*, 2008) explores the gender dimensions of mental health problems. Cohen and Mullender (2002) discuss gender in the context of groupwork. Christie (*Men and Social Work: Theories and Practices*, 2001) also provides an interesting set of readings on the subject of men and social work, while Segal (*Slow Motion: Changing Masculinities, Changing Men*, 2007) is an important source for understanding men in society in general. Lister (*Citizenship: Feminist Perspectives*, 2003) presents an important account of feminist perspectives on citizenship. Scott, Treas and Richards (*The Blackwell Companion to the Sociology of Families*, 2007) offer a very helpful set of discussions of the family.

General texts on feminism and gender include: Banyard, (*The Equality Illusion: The Truth about Women and Men Today*, 2011); Fine (*Delusions of Gender: The Real Science Behind Sex Differences*, 2011); Pilcher and Whelehan (*50 Key Concepts in Gender Studies*, 2004), and Richardson and Robinson (*Introducing Gender and Women's Studies*, 2007),

Thompson (*Effective Communication: A Guide for the People Professions*, 2011b) discusses gender issues in relation to communication and language. Riches ('Gender', 2002) focuses on gender issues in relation to loss and grief, as do Doka and Martin (*Grieving Beyond Gender: Understanding the Ways Women Mourn*, 2010).

ETHNICITY AND RACISM

Introduction

The United Kingdom, it is often said, is a multicultural society. That is, it is composed of a variety of ethnic groups, each with different characteristics and patterns. How important this is for social work forms the major analytical focus of this chapter. Bullock and Trombley define ethnicity as: 'communal characteristics: lingual, ancestral, regional, religious etc., which are seen to be the basis of distinctive identity' (2000, p. 285). The term is particularly significant when used to describe minority groups within a society – that is, ethnic minorities. It is often forgotten that all people are 'ethnic' – that is, belong to a cultural group – and so it is both inaccurate and misleading to refer to members of ethnic minorities as 'ethnics' or 'ethnic people'. This implies that to be a member of the ethnic majority is 'normal' and so members of ethnic minorities are by definition deviant or 'abnormal'. This, as we shall see below, is a form of racism.

But ethnicity is only one part of the situation; it is by no means the whole story. Ethnicity implies difference, whereas the dominant notion social workers encounter is that of deficit. Members of ethnic minorities are often perceived as inferior and are thus subject to discrimination and hence oppression. Ethnic minority groups are presented, ideologically, as biologically different from and, by implication, inferior to, the ethnic majority. In this way, ethnic difference (characterized by solidarity, shared values and positively valued cultural identity) is constructed as racial

rized by exclusion, marginalization and oppression). It
int to see ethnicity and race in conjunction, as the
)f ethnicity are used as a political weapon to reinforce
ninant majority, in so far as these differences are seen
ie ethnocentric norm.
railure to recognize this covert shift from ethnicity to race serves to
mask racism and its subtle influences. In short, the United Kingdom, the
United States and other western countries are indeed multicultural, but to
focus exclusively on cultural or ethnic patterns without taking account of
'race' is indeed a naïve mistake. Race is not a biological category, it is a
process – a social and political process whereby ethnic differences are
translated into pseudo-biological racial deficits. In this way, the seeds of
racism are sown. Discrimination against black and ethnic minority peoples
is legitimated on the basis of assumed racial inferiority. This is a point to
which I shall return below.

Social workers dealing with a wide range of ethnic communities therefore need to be aware of ethnic differences (ethnically sensitive social
work) and the commonalities across minority groups – that is, oppression,
discrimination and relative powerlessness (anti-racist social work). This
chapter seeks to establish a clearer understanding of the racial dimension
of social work and take steps towards the development of an anti-racist
social work practice base. The first step towards this must be a clarification
of the central concept of racism.

What is racism?

Burke and Harrison define racism in the following terms:

> Racism is a multidimensional and complex system of power and powerless-
> ness. It is a process through which powerful groups, using deterministic
> belief systems and structures in society, are able to dominate. It operates
> at micro and macro levels, is developed through specific cognitions and
> actions, and perpetuated and sustained through policies and procedures of
> social systems and institutions. This can be seen in the differential outcomes
> for less powerful groups in accessing services in the health and welfare, edu-
> cation, housing and the legal and criminal justice systems.
>
> (Burke and Harrison, 2000, p. 283)

This is a most helpful definition that incorporates some very important
elements. It is very compatible with PCS analysis, in so far as it shows that

racism is not simply a matter of individual prejudice
plex and multi-layered than that. Another long-st
offered by Chakrabarti when he argued that:

> Racism is, first a set of beliefs or a way of thinkin
> identified on the basis of real or imagined biologi
> colour, for example) are thought necessarily to possess other characteristics
> that are viewed in a negative light ... It is rooted in the belief that certain
> groups, identified as 'races', 'ethnic minorities' or by some more abusive
> label, share characteristics such as attitudes or abilities and a propensity
> to certain behaviour. The assumption is made that every person, whether
> man, woman or child, classified as belonging to such a group, is possessed
> of all these characteristics.
>
> (Chakrabarti, 1990, p. 15)

This definition includes a number of key elements:

Beliefs and values are a basic part of racism – that is, racism is an ideology.

1   It relates to 'real or imagined biological characteristics'. Racism is
    therefore socially constructed rather than biologically given (Soydan
    and Williams, 1998).

2   Racism is a negative term: it carries strong negative connotations and
    is used as a form of abuse (and, by extension, discrimination and
    oppression).

3   Stereotypical assumptions are used to sustain this negativity and thus
    to maintain the dominance, power and privilege of the white
    majority.

A simpler and more well-known definition is that of Katz (1978): 'prejudice
plus power'. This is useful, in so far as it points out that racism is more than
just a matter of personal prejudice, but is indeed a much wider issue. However, this definition and the approach of Katz in general have been discredited, as we shall see in our discussion below on Race Awareness Training.

One important point to recognize is that, regardless of which definition we may favour, racism remains a serious social problem and a significant source of oppression for significant numbers of people, as the
comments from Stiglitz, writing in a US context, exemplify:

> Thus, on average, being black reduces employment opportunities
> substantially, and ore so for ex-offenders. These effects can present

he's Black, brown, yellow or green' ... . Such a perspective is, however, one of privilege, for those who are racially oppressed know that their skin colour is often of profound significance. Even when white people can see the racial disadvantages experienced by black people, they are frequently unable to see that this also means that they themselves are privileged by their whiteness, and that racial advantage is not simply the product of individual racist acts, but of a whole system of racial hierarchy.

(Bryson, 1999, p. 52)

Similarly, Sivanandan (1991) was right to point out the weakness inherent in the Scarman Report of 1982 (into 'race' riots) which also laid too great a stress on the **P** level. He puts this point across quite strongly in the following passage:

Basically, Scarman said there is no institutional racism but there is racial prejudice. He took away the objective facts of institutional racism and made them subjective. So that what we had to tackle was not the system, not the power, not the police on the streets, not the immigration officers who examined my sister to see if she was a virgin. What we had to change was the immigration officer's mind, so that he would not dislike my sister. That is nonsense.

(Sivanandan, 1991, p. 42)

PCS analysis also alerts us to the fact that racism is not necessarily intentional. In reflecting dominant cultural values or carrying out routine institutional practices, we may actually be perpetrating acts of racism unwittingly. For example, working on the stereotypical premise that Asian families 'look after their own' may prevent Asian clients from receiving the level of support they require. Although this may not be racist in intention, it is none the less racist in effect or outcome, and is therefore likely to be experienced as oppressive.

Voice of experience 4.1
_____

I had always thought of racism as something intentional based on people's prejudices, but the equality and diversity course I attended made it clear there is much more to it than that. It helped me understand that if minority ethnic groups are disadvantaged by an action or a policy then that amounts to racism. Racism isn't just about intentions, it's also about outcomes. *Jill, a social worker in a family support team*

...losely to the important concept of 'institutional racism' which ...d in the Macpherson report (into a racist murder) as the:

> c.. .ve failure of an organization to provide an appropriate and profes-
> sional service to people because of their colour, culture or ethnic origin. It
> can be seen or detected in processes, attitudes and behaviour which amount
> to discrimination through unwitting prejudice, ignorance, thoughtlessness
> and racist stereotyping which disadvantage minority ethnic people.
>
> (Macpherson, 1999, p. 4)

Racism can be, and often is, deeply ingrained in the culture of an organization and will therefore often manifest itself even if individuals are not deliberately perpetrating overtly racist acts. Institutional racism therefore refers to racism at the cultural and structural levels. It is a concept that reinforces the importance of recognizing the complexity of discrimination and oppression and not simply reducing them to personal prejudice.

In this respect, and indeed many others, racism can be seen to parallel sexism, in so far as the processes which underpin both sexism and racism have much in common. Thus, in seeking to understand racism, looking to our knowledge of sexism can help us move forward. However, we must none the less avoid the mistake of allowing the similarities to distract us from the significant differences (for example, the role of sexuality in sexism or the legacy of imperialism in racism).

Racism serves to 'pathologize' black individuals and families, to present them as inferior to, and therefore less worthy than, their white counterparts. This tendency is also visible in social work and therefore has major implications for practice. As Robinson comments:

> Many social work texts paint crude cultural stereotypes of black families.
> The 'norm' against which black families are, implicitly or explicitly,
> judged is white. The norm presents a myth of the normal family as
> nuclear, middle class and heterosexual. Black families are seen as strange,
> different and inferior.
>
> (Robinson, 2002, p. 91)

Of course, it would be a reductionist oversimplification to assume that this applies to all interactions between social workers and black families. However, Robinson's point presents an important warning that social workers need to be very wary of allowing dominant cultural representations of black families (fuelled in large part by distorted media representations) to seduce them into relying on distorted perceptions of black individuals, families and communities.

Practice focus 4.1

Jill was a newly qualified social worker in a child care team. At an allocation meeting she was very interested in the case of the Bhogal family where there had been suspicions of neglect. Jill therefore expressed a willingness to take the case. However, to her great surprise and consternation, her team leader, Mike, commented that it would be better suited to a more experienced worker 'considering this is a black family'. When challenged about this, Mike found it very difficult to explain or justify his remarks. He could only reiterate that the case needed a more experienced worker. Jill therefore remained concerned about Mike's apparent negative assumptions about black families.

Such negative stereotypes serve to reinforce the process of pathologizing individuals, families and cultures who 'deviate' from the dominant white norm. This is one example among many of the implications of racism for social work policy, theory and practice. We shall return to this topic later in this chapter. First, however, we need to consider some further dimensions of ethnicity.

Language, nation and region

There are, of course, close links between factors associated with one's language, national or regional identity and ethnic groupings. A key unifying concept in this area is that of culture – what can be defined at its simplest as shared ways of seeing, thinking and doing. Cultural values and norms differ across regions and nations, and also within or across linguistic groups. Indeed, it has long been recognized that language is a central part of culture. As Carter and Aitchison comment:

> The character and vitality of a culture is to a large extent language-dependent. Language helps to preserve traditions, shapes modes of perception, and profoundly influences patterns of social intercourse and behaviour.
>
> (Carter and Aitchison, 1986, p. 1)

They go on to quote Mandelbaum (1949, p. 162): 'No two languages are ever sufficiently similar to be considered as representing the same social reality' (ibid.).

On this basis, the language or languages one speaks (and, by implication, through which one conducts one's own social interactions) have a profound impact on the way in which we experience our existence – the medium through which we make sense of our world and construct our reality.

This will be very significant where the social worker is from a different linguistic background from the client or group with which he or she is working. This may be where languages of ethnic minority groups are involved, for example, Urdu or Gujarati, and the appropriate use of an interpreter is likely to be needed. The legislative base also requires practitioners to demonstrate some degree of linguistic sensitivity – for example, in terms of the Children Act 1989 or the requirement, under the Mental Health Act 1983, to interview 'in an appropriate manner', although it must be acknowledged that such issues may frequently be neglected.

Making sure that members of ethnic minorities have the opportunity to communicate their needs, wishes and feelings is, of course, part and parcel of anti-racist practice. However, there are other cross-linguistic situations which are not so directly associated with racism – although ethnocentrism does tend to feature. I am referring to bilingual nations, such as Canada and Wales. As Drakeford and Morris point out: 'Almost every state in Europe is at least bilingual, in the sense of having more than one indigenous language, as well as languages spoken by migrants from other places' (1998, p. 93). To take Wales as an example, there are over half a million people within the principality who speak the Welsh language (2001 census figures). Most of these people also speak English but it should be noted that, for very many, English is a 'second language'. For dealing with sensitive matters, perhaps of an emotional nature, communicating in one's first language is very much to be preferred.

Practice focus 4.2

Ceri was a social worker in a family placement team. She regularly used Welsh as a means of communication with clients and colleagues, including foster carers. She often felt uncomfortable about placing Welsh-speaking children with foster carers who spoke only English but a shortage of foster carers often meant that choices were not available. However, the matter was particularly significant in the case of one eight-year-old girl who, when placed with English-speaking foster carers, began to disclose incidents of sexual abuse that had occurred when she had stayed with her aunt and uncle. However, she very quickly 'clammed up', and it was only when Ceri visited her and communicated in Welsh that she felt able to discuss some very painful and distressing experiences.

This point has been recognized by the Care Council for Wales who have produced a multimedia training resource, entitled *They All Speak English Anyway* (referring to a sadly not uncommon tendency on some people's part to dismiss the significance of the Welsh language) (Care Council for Wales, 2010). In Wales a client has the basic right to choose the language of interaction with the social work agency. It is important, therefore, to ensure that linguistic issues are addressed, particularly in bilingual communities. Failure to do so could act as an extra layer of oppression by forcing Welsh speakers (or indeed speakers of any non-dominant language – the issue is not confined to Wales) to communicate from a position of relative weakness (see Davies, 2009 for a helpful discussion of the complex issues involved). Furthermore, Bellin (1994) also argues that it is necessary, in working with bilingual individuals, families and communities, to give due regard to both languages:

> Social work practice needs to recognize that the bilingual Welsh-speaker is just as much an integrated whole person as a mono-lingual. This means that it is an unacceptable short-cut to rely on just one language for intervention or rendering of service.
>
> (Bellin, 1994, p. 116)

To take no account of a client's first language can be seen as devaluing that language and indeed the culture of which it forms part and the personal identity of the client(s) concerned. This is an example of 'ethnocentrism', the tendency to take one's own cultural or ethnic standpoint for granted without reference to other perspectives, thus imposing one's own definitions as the 'norm'.

One notable manifestation of ethnocentrism in this context is to equate 'British' with 'English', as if Wales and Scotland were simply regions of England. This is captured in Morgan's comment in which he refers to: 'that notorious entry in the Encyclopaedia Britannica – in which were encapsulated all the humiliation and patronizing indifference which helped to launch the modern nationalist movement in the principality – "for Wales, see England"' (1982, p. 3). There are clear implications here for anti-discriminatory social work practice. Social workers need to be sensitive to the culture and values of not only black and ethnic minority communities, but also national, regional and linguistic groups. To ignore these factors is to ignore major aspects of the client's experience, values and social location and thus fall foul of ethnocentrism.

The concept of ethnocentrism is a useful one, in so far as it takes us beyond the individual level of personal prejudice and emphasizes the role of culture and thus the social dimension. However, this in itself has

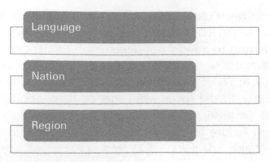

Figure 4.1 Language, nation and region

limitations, as it takes no account of the structural level. One longstanding approach to these issues which does have a structural basis is that of Hechter (1999) who draws on the concept of 'internal colonialism', the idea that the Celtic nations can be seen to function as internal colonies within the United Kingdom, serving the interests of the ruling (capitalist) groups.

Harris, in a paper discussing anti-racist social work, drew important parallels between the oppression of black people and the historic treatment of the Welsh. He comments:

> Language is the main medium by means of which culture is transmitted. It is also the mechanism which enables the functions of conceiving, defining, refining and articulating ideas. Therefore if cultural hegemony is the objective, it is not surprising that bilingualism could not be tolerated either, as in the case of the Welsh the possession of that ability would have placed them in an advantageous position. The Welsh would have enjoyed the flexibility and facility of operating within and between two language mediums, while still retaining their cultural autonomy. In contrast the English ruling class would have been constrained, since being monolingual, they would have been unable to enter directly into the consciousness of the Welsh. Colonized people and immigrants are often encouraged by means of bribes or coercion to adopt the language of their oppressors.
>
> (Harris, 1991, pp. 138–9)

A key term here is 'cultural hegemony'. Anti-discriminatory social work should play no part in the maintenance of such dominance, with its implied oppression of cultural or linguistic minorities.

The example given here has been that of Wales, but the same issues can be seen to apply to a wider range of peoples in a wide variety of places in which social work is practised. Negative and derogatory stereotypes of Irish people is an example which springs readily to mind. Indeed, Garrett

(2004) is right to emphasize that there is more to racism than what he calls the 'black/white binary', as there is a long history of anti-Irish racism that also needs to be considered.

Key point 4.1

Over the years there has been a tendency for people to oversimplify racism. If we are to ensure that certain groups or individuals are not disadvantaged because of one or more aspects of their ethnicity, then we need to be tuned in to subtleties and complexities involved.

There is therefore a need for social workers to give due consideration to the issues of national, regional and linguistic identity as they apply as aspects of ethnicity in the locality in which they work. Without this there is a danger that an insensitive social work practice can contribute further to the oppression of 'cultural hegemony', rather than play a part in reducing the alienation and disempowerment it engenders.

The implications for social work

One very clear implication to be drawn from the literature on racism and social work is that traditional social work has seriously neglected the racial dimension of the social problems it seeks to tackle and the impact of racism on ethnic minority communities.

It even goes beyond this to the point where social work practice can itself be racist, whether by acts of omission or commission, whether deliberate or unwitting. In the past thirty years or so, social work has had to re-evaluate its assumptions about race, culture and ethnicity and to become more alert to the presence and impact of racism. This is not to say that social workers are 'racists' who deliberately try to short-change their black clients – that would be to confuse the **P** level with the wider levels of **C** and **S**. The actions of social workers need to be seen in their wider cultural and structural context, but we should not make the mistake of assuming that the **C** and/or **S** levels determine our actions at the **P** level.

In one sense it is hard to believe that decent social workers committed to being helpful could contribute so strongly to discrimination and oppression. However, it needs to be recognized that we are part of a wider framework which reflects power and privilege differences and which hinges on social divisions. This therefore brings us back to the point emphasized earlier, namely: if we are not part of the solution, we must be part of the problem. While our actions are not *determined* by wider forces, they can, if we are not careful, reinforce those wider forces. For example, by uncritically relying on racist stereotypes, we are not only reflecting the cultural level, but also reproducing it.

Racism, like all discrimination, is often unintentional and operates via acts of omission as well as commission, and so the excuse that we were not aware of 'the problem' is not a valid one. When we become aware of the racism inherent in the culture and institutions of social work (the **C** and **S** levels), our own actions (the **P** level) will either reflect, reinforce and consolidate such racism, or may go at least some small way to challenging and undermining it. There can be no neutral territory.

One way in which racism manifests itself in social work is in the over-representation of black people in 'control' situations and under-representation in 'care' situations.

The power of the social worker can at times be considerable. Where this power is premised on racist assumptions, unwitting stereotypes or other such aspects of institutional racism, the disservice to black or minority ethnic clients is likely to be of major proportions.

The mental health field is a good example of this. Morgan et al. (2006) report that diagnoses of psychotic conditions can be up to 18 times more frequent for African-Caribbean people than for white people. The same authors point out that African-Caribbean people who experience psychotic conditions are also much more likely to come into contact with mental health services through what they call 'adversarial routes' (via the police or compulsory admissions). The findings presented in this research report raise the question of what role is racism playing in this situation. There are (at least) three main ways in which racism could be a factor:

1 There are problems of diagnosis and response to mental health crises, with the danger that racist assumptions (based on stereotypes and a lack of understanding of how emotions are characteristically expressed in certain cultural groups) are influencing how African-Caribbean people are being dealt with within mental health services.

2 Stresses and strains and possible traumatic experiences associated with: (i) migration and its consequences in terms of upheaval (but recognizing that most African-Caribbean people living in the United Kingdom will have been born here and are not therefore immigrants); (ii) direct, overt experiences of racism (abuse, violence and so on); (iii) more subtle, indirect experiences of racism (for example, institutional

discrimination); and (iv) poverty, deprivation, poor housing and other social problems which African-Caribbean people are more likely to encounter.

3   A combination of the above (and quite possibly other factors too).

Being aware of the dangers involved in (1) is an important step towards ethnically sensitive practice – a practice which seeks to avoid the pitfalls of a distorted diagnosis based on an inadequate appreciation of cultural patterns, values and norms. This is a *necessary* condition for anti-racism but, as we shall see below in our discussion of multiculturalism, it is not a *sufficient* condition that is, it is a step in the right direction, but it is not enough on its own.

Being aware of (2) should help us to develop a fuller, more holistic picture of racism in particular and discrimination in general with a fuller appreciation of the sociological aspects of discrimination – again reinforcing the need to move away from perspectives on discrimination that are limited to individual prejudice.

Inappropriate use of powers under the Mental Health Act 1983 is an easy trap for social workers to fall into if they are not sufficiently aware of the racial dimension of psychiatry, their own potential for unwittingly reinforcing racist assumptions and practices and those of other professionals within the mental health field. It is to be hoped, then, that the mistakes of the past in relation to race, culture and mental health can be avoided by social workers (and, indeed, other mental health workers) with a more sophisticated understanding of the complex workings of discriminatory processes in society in general and in professional practice in particular.

Similar issues arise in relation to the over-representation of black children in care (Owen and Statham, 2009). We can but speculate as to the precise reasons for such over-representation, but these are likely to include:

- a lack of effective preventative work due to the reluctance or inability of white social workers to work with black families;

- the reluctance of black families to engage in preventative work due to their mistrust of (potentially) racist social work organizations; and

- the tendency to pathologize black families (Collins, 2000).

These examples of the over-representation of black people in 'control' situations are paralleled by an equivalent under-representation in 'caring' or supportive services. Numerous sources refer to the relative neglect of black and minority ethnic people in terms of the provision of supportive social services (Robinson, 2008).

Social work has long been recognized as a mixture of care and control and, to a large extent, the two elements represent two sides of the same coin (Thompson, 2015b). However, the situation in relation to black and ethnic minority clients is that there is a distinct imbalance. The control element is very much to the fore, while the caring element features far less than is the case with white clients.

What this demonstrates is that racism not only acts as a barrier to good practice but actually 'uses' social work as a vehicle for further discrimination and oppression. In the wake of the Macpherson report, there has been a major focus on institutional racism in the police force. However, we should certainly not be complacent enough to assume that social work is free of such problems (Penketh, 2000).

This relates to the point made in Chapter 1 – that good practice must be anti-discriminatory practice; a social work which is unaware of its potential for discrimination and oppression is a dangerous social work. These issues are particularly pertinent to the process of assessment – gauging the nature and extent of the problems and the resources available or needed. There are two main sets of issues involved. First, there is the cultural dimension. There is a danger that assessment will be based on dominant white norms without adequate attention being paid to cultural differences. Failure to take such differences into account will not only distort, and thereby invalidate, the basis of the assessment but will also serve to alienate clients by devaluing their culture (Thompson, 2009b).

But this means more than distinguishing between white culture and 'black culture' for there is no one single black culture (as, indeed, there is no one 'white' culture). Black cultures are many and varied and to ignore this is to operate at a stereotypical level, to oversimplify a complex picture. Ethnically sensitive social work involves developing at least a basic understanding of local minority ethnic communities and cultures. Social work assessment needs to be based on understanding and analysis rather than ignorance and assumptions.

Parekh (2008) emphasizes the importance of recognizing cultural differences as part of a commitment to valuing diversity. In terms of other cultures, he argues that:

> One does not merely tolerate or even respect them from a difference, but values and cherishes them, and wishes them well. When they flourish and develop their characteristic forms of excellence, one benefits just as their members do. The diversity of perspectives and their sympathetic and critical interaction is a universal human good, which we have a collective interest in promoting.
>
> (Parekh, 2008, p. 227)

And, of course, the cultural pluralism is further extend
a significant and growing proportion of black peopl
cent and 87 per cent, according to ethnic group – S
were born in Britain and have therefore been brought
ence of the culture of their parents and the domina
transmitted by the media, the education system and so on.

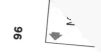

Black communities are therefore different, both from each other and from the white majority – this is the dimension of ethnicity. What social work assessment also needs to take into account is what black communities have in common – their experience of racism. Prevatt Goldstein writes of the dangers of:

> an over-reliance on cultural, religious interpretations which can assume cultures are static and homogenous and overlook the individual, condone oppressive elements within cultures and religions, and substitute cultural solutions for challenging oppressive interactions and structures.
>
> (Prevatt Goldstein, 2008, p. 418)

Once again, then, we see that awareness of cultural differences is important but it is no substitute for awareness of racism and the need to challenge it. Prevatt Goldstein goes on to argue that there needs to be a willingness to identify and name racism:

> This naming of the daily experiences of racism and the powerful structures of racism can be demoralizing and disempowering if it is situated only in negative experiences of being black and in a context where racism is being experienced or challenged in isolation. The implications for social work practice include challenging all forms of racism as well as the placement of black children where they will not be isolated in their experience, a reduction in the isolation of black people in day care, residential provision, service delivery, decision-making forums and the development of groups for black service users and workers.
>
> (Prevatt Goldstein, 2008, p. 420)

Practice focus 4.3

Steve was a very competent student on placement in a specialist team for older people. In response to a referral from a local GP, he was asked to undertake an assessment of Mrs Jordan, a woman of West Indian origin. He set about his task with enthusiasm and did a lot of background reading. He interviewed

▶

s Jordan on three separate occasions and was very thorough in gathering information about her life, her background and her needs, paying particular attention to the cultural aspects of the situation. Steve's practice teacher congratulated him on the quality of his work and his success in working in an ethnically sensitive way. However, she had to point out to him that, despite this, he had failed to address issues of racism. He had not taken into account what part racism had played in shaping her current circumstances or how racism may affect her current and future needs. His work was therefore ethnically sensitive but not anti-racist.

It is perhaps easier and less uncomfortable for us to take on board cultural diversity without going a step further and acknowledging racism and the need to challenge it. There are times when we can indulge in seeing the rich variety of cultural patterns as a contribution to social life, an 'entertainment' to make white lives more interesting but without also recognizing the disadvantages and discrimination ethnic minority communities experience – as I put it earlier we need to appreciate adversity as well as diversity.

Cultural awareness (or 'cultural competence' as it is often called these days) promotes ethnically sensitive practice and thus helps to avoid the problems of devaluing minority cultures or seeing them as inferior to white culture and thereby alienating the people who share those cultures. This is a valuable step forward but, it is also necessary to take the further step of recognizing potential elements of racism in ourselves (reflecting the culture we were brought up in), our practice and our agencies. It is only then that we can move towards anti-racist practice.

Voice of experience 4.2

I have found that many people are much more culturally aware than used to be the case in the past, and that's good to see, but sadly there are still quite a few people I meet who seem to be wearing blinkers. They see the world through the lens of their own culture and don't seem to recognize that their culture is just one amongst many. So, we've made some progress, but we still have a long way to go. *Rashid, a workforce development officer*

One aspect of the relationship between racism and social work which is often not appreciated is that the foundations of anti-racist social work are actually enshrined in legislation. Over the years there has been a number of legislative provisions that have included the need to address racism and associated matters (the Equality Act 2010 being the latest). But, of course, it would be naïve to assume that such a broad legislative statement could ensure a firm foundation for anti-racist practice. A tighter and much more specific set of policy guidelines and regulations would be necessary to provide such a baseline for anti-discriminatory policies which can readily be translated into practice. In addition, however, over twenty-five years ago Ahmad made the important point that:

> No legislation alone can make social workers anti-racist. Much depends on how they interpret the laws or even abuse them to reinforce racism. Much also depends on how legislations are used as a tool to tackle racism in social work.
>
> (Ahmad, 1990, p. 5)

Of course, this remains as true now as when the point was originally made. As I have already indicated, anti-discriminatory practice means much more than seeking legal compliance with anti-discrimination legislation.

Racism is a powerful force in society. It subjects one portion of society – black and minority ethnic groups – to oppression, degradation and discrimination on the grounds that they are deemed to be inferior, by virtue of biology and/or culture, to the white majority. As Frazer puts it:

> Racism is an abuse of power. It means treating people as inferior or less capable on the grounds of their race, colour or ethnic difference. It results in discrimination against people and the denial of their fundamental rights.
>
> (Frazer, 2001, p. 140)

When we consider this carefully, it becomes clear that this situation has major implications for social work in terms of policies, theory base, practice, training, recruitment and management. Space does not permit a detailed analysis of these issues (see 'Further resources' at the end of the chapter), but I shall return later in this chapter to focus specifically on some of the practice implications.

Having drawn, albeit rather sketchily, some of the links between racism and social work, let us now consider some of the factors leading to the development of contemporary approaches to anti-racism.

The anti-racist response

Although there have been black communities in Britain for centuries, it was in the late 1940s and early 1950s that race relations issues began to take on increasingly major significance as a result of specific historical developments at that time.

In the years following the end of the Second World War there were labour shortages which, it was felt, would hold back the promised new age of prosperity and post-war reconstruction. It was therefore felt necessary to seek out new sources of labour to expand the workforce and thus sustain economic development. The New Commonwealth countries were seen as a rich seam of potential workers and so these areas were targeted for an intensive advertising and promotional campaign to persuade possible recruits to emigrate to Britain. This campaign was largely successful and led to a rise in Britain's black population.

However, what this campaign did not emphasize was that the jobs available were the lowest paid and the least popular. It was also not made clear that no additional, health or educational facilities would be provided. In particular, the failure to consider housing need exacerbated the existing housing shortage which meant that the vast majority of the invited immigrants lived in very poor quality conditions in seriously overcrowded accommodation.

The link between race and class became strongly established as black people very quickly became over-represented at the lower levels of Britain's socioeconomic class system (the relationship between class and race is an important one, and one to which I shall return later). It was not long before black people were seen not as the victims of poverty, inadequate housing and so on, but as a significant part of the cause of such problems.

An attitude of racial superiority among the white 'hosts' was instrumental in translating the structurally based problems experienced by black people into matters of personal failing, weakness or inadequacy – poverty caused by 'not working hard enough', poor housing by having 'lower standards' and so on. The next step was to blame black people for the problems experienced by white people: 'they take our jobs', and 'they cause trouble'. This was the emergence of racism on a much wider scale than ever before. The focus was not on the problems of black people brought about by the Government's poorly thought-out migrant labour policy, but rather on black people as a problem. This pattern persists to this day: the problem of racism is conveniently reframed as the problem of race.

An early response to this situation was the develop[ ] known as the assimilationist approach. The propo[ ] black people should integrate as far as possible i[ ] society so that they did not attract hostility by b[ ] short, the answer to white hostility was seen as [ ] 'white' in all but skin colour. Once again we see an[ ] superiority – adopting white norms is seen as advantageous to black peo-ple. The loss of ethnicity and cultural 'belongingness' is not considered important and the development of positive black identities is obstructed. According to this model, the best that a black person can become is 'almost white'. Penketh summarizes the situation as follows:

> Assimilationist perspectives are based on the belief in the cultural and racial superiority of white society and the associated belief that black groups should be absorbed into the indigenous homogeneous culture. That is, they are expected to adopt the British 'way of life' and not to undermine the social and ideological bases of the dominant culture. Integrationist perspectives also subscribe to assumptions of cultural superiority, and therefore place the responsibility on black communities to learn 'new customs' and ways of behaving in order to be accepted by the indigenous population.
>
> (Penketh, 2000, p. 24)

A significant aspect of this approach is the attempt to seek to minimize differences between black and white. The assimilationist approach is there-fore characterized as 'colour blind'. In social work this amounts to ignoring the different needs of ethnic minority groups (brought about in no small part by the impact of racism) and treating them in a uniform, undifferenti-ated way – a far cry from the notion of valuing and affirming diversity.

A very different but similarly problematic approach which follows a different logic is that of multiculturalism. The emphasis here is not on minimizing differences between black and white but rather on cultural diversity. The differences between white 'main-stream' culture and the various black cultures are given due regard, in theory at least, and such differences can actually be celebrated as enriching the cultural life of all. Ethnicity is positively valued and diversity is presented as a potential ben-efit, rather than a problem. Up to a point, this is a significant improve-ment on the assimilationist position, as it does avoid the problems of sweeping ethnic differences under the carpet. However, it does not go far enough and, albeit unintentionally, can actually allow racism to persist, but in a more respectable form (but see Parekh, 2006, for a discussion of the value of multiculturalism).

.oach which did not ignore power was that of Race Awareness or 'RAT' as it became known. RAT was based on Katz's (1978) .ion of racism as 'prejudice plus power'. However, the sort of power which it referred was that of individuals by virtue of their job or status ivanandan, 1991, p. 43), rather than social or political power on a wider structural basis. A further problem with this approach was that its attempts to tackle racial prejudice were based on an aggressive, confrontational approach that turned out to be counterproductive, partly because it led to a high level of anxiety and defensiveness which blocked learning (Thompson, 2009b) and partly because, as Husband (1986) put it at the time this approach was in favour: 'Race awareness training can produce a socially competent non-racist performance; it does not produce an anti-racist practice' (1986, p. 11).

Practice focus 4.4

Karen was an experienced trainer who frequently ran courses on equality issues. On one particular course she was concerned that Phil, one of the participants, became very distressed and anxious when the subject of racism was raised. Consequently, during the coffee break she had a word with him to check that he was all right. He apologized for possibly disrupting the course, but he was experiencing very painful memories of a course he had attended some ten years earlier where a highly confrontational approach had been adopted. For Phil, and so many others, the experience had left him feeling confused and anxious and had encouraged him to adopt a defensive attitude towards the whole subject area.

These various approaches to 'race relations' have all failed to address the central feature of the problem, namely racism, premised on:

1 The hostility of many white people to black;

2 The assumed superiority which legitimates this; and

3 The unequal distribution of power, privilege, resources and life chances which such hostility sustains.

In the early days of social work's growing commitment to anti-racist practice Roys made a comment that still applies today:

The difficulties faced by the black population are the result not only of migration and differences in culture and language but also of living in a society which is hostile to black people, denies them equal life chances and can expose them to enormous material and psychological pressure. The clients of social services present with not only linguistic and cultural complexities but also with the profound effects of racism.

(Roys, 1988, p. 221)

Modern anti-racism dismisses the oppression and 'cultural imperialism' of assimilationism and transcends the cultural pluralism of multiculturalism. It recognizes the structural basis of racism and how this underpins the cultural and personal dimensions of racial discrimination.

How anti-racism can possibly be made a reality in social work practice will be discussed below, but we must first clarify, to a certain extent at least, the relationships between race and class on the one hand, and race and gender on the other.

Race, class and gender

The presence of black communities in Britain is an issue not only of race but also of class. The primary reason for the initial migration of black people was the capitalist economy's need to boost its workforce – to extend the working class. Also, as was noted above, the jobs that were available to be filled were low paid and of low status and thus at the bottom of the class hierarchy.

There are close links between race and class. Indeed, racism can be seen as an ideology which divides the working class by setting worker against worker and thereby contributes to the continuance of capitalism by discouraging working-class solidarity. However, it is a mistake to see the social division of race as a subcategory of class. Class and race articulate together; that is, they are interrelated. Williams captures this point when he argues that:

> race is defined not as a 'natural' or biological attribute but as a socially and historically constructed concept by which members of society endow skin color variations, which have no intrinsic meaning, with meanings that reinforce a hierarchy of privilege and power in society. Class is defined as a system of stratification in which unequal allocation of resources and opportunity for social advancement is supported by cultural myths that naturalize inequality. Although these concepts are conceptually distinct, they are related in interesting and complicated ways. ... [C]lass issues are often concealed in racially coded language and meanings. Racial stereotypes are frequently used to reinforce a system of class inequality while class stereotypes are used to reinforce a racial hierarchy.

(Williams, 2000, p. 215)

Furthermore, Wilkinson (2005) makes the point that class inequalities have the effect of differences in ethnicity, religion or language – which might otherwise be easily accepted and not seen as significant – becoming targets for social prejudices. If class inequalities were not so great, he argues, issues of social superiority and social inferiority would receive far less attention and cause far less friction.

In short, racism should not be seen in a vacuum, separate from class and economic factors, but nor should it be seen as simply a by-product or subcategory of the social division of class (Roberts, 2011).

This parallels the debate in the previous chapter about the relationship between capitalism and patriarchy. But what we now need to consider is the third aspect of the class, race, gender triangle – the relationship between race and gender.

Feminism, in its earlier formulations at least, has been characterized by an emphasis on the common oppression of women, the shared experience of 'sisterhood'. However, the appropriateness of such an emphasis has increasingly been called into question. It is argued that the tendency to focus almost exclusively on the commonalities of women's experience leads to a disregard for significant differences between women, particularly in terms of race. Ramazanoglu (1989) extends this argument to include other divisions between women – for example, sexual orientation – and this reinforces the critique of an oversimplified analysis of women's experience of oppression. Ramazanoglu also points to the class dimension inherent in the attack on white feminism when she underlines the highly educated middle-class ethos of the movement (1989, p. 129), which no doubt further fuelled the anger of the critics.

Key point 4.2

It is essential to recognize that forms of discrimination interact with one another. They are not discrete, separate entities. We need to have a holistic understanding of how discrimination operates and how we can counter it.

The theme of anti-sexism needing to take on board issues of anti-racism has been a recurring one. It features in work stretching back over four decades, ranging from hooks (1982, 1986) through to Segal (2007) and Cole (2011). However, there is clearly a growing awareness of the need for feminism to incorporate an anti-racist perspective and the implications of this are a feature of feminist and anti-racist scholarship – see, for example, Collins (2000).

It has been recognized that it is not simply a matter of 'tagging on' racism to sexism as the complex interactions of the two need to be explored and clarified (Mullender, 2008). The dynamic interplay of class, race and gender is indeed complex and multifaceted (see *Promoting Equality* for a fuller discussion of these issues). And, indeed, it will continue to be so, as this is an ongoing dynamic – historically variable and far beyond a simple once-and-for-all solution. Although very complex, this is an area where social workers need to have at least a basic grasp of the fundamental issues in order to construct an adequate theoretical basis for anti-discriminatory practice.

Towards anti-racist practice

Distilling the principles of anti-racist social work is by no means an easy task, especially as this is a rapidly changing area and one prone to considerable political conflict and widely differing sets of values. None the less, the remainder of this chapter is an attempt to crystallize some of the basic tenets of anti-racist social work as I see it. Given the nature of the subject matter, this attempt can be neither definitive nor comprehensive. The aim is to inform, raise consciousness and thus promote further study and debate rather than to provide 'the answer'.

1 The first step towards anti-racism is to recognize and eradicate any tendencies towards racism that may be present in our own practice (for example, as a result of relying on stereotypes). This is not a RAT-style guilt trip, but rather an acknowledgement (in line with PCS analysis) of the structural and cultural influences on our behaviour and attitudes. If we are not sensitive to these issues, if we do not attempt to swim against the tide of racism, then we will be carried along by the strong current, knowingly or otherwise. Failing to act against racism could be seen as in itself a form of unintentional racism that involves condoning significant inequality and injustice.

2 For many years now there has been considerable rhetoric about anti-racism and the notion of equal opportunities in general. There is therefore a danger that anti-racism remains at a rhetorical level only. It is much more comfortable for people to deal with it at this level without actually engaging with the issues. There must be a real commitment

to tackling some difficult and painful issues. The rhetoric is only of value if it is backed up by reality.

3   Social work with black and minority ethnic clients must operate on the basis of cultural difference and not deficit. All steps must be taken to ensure that assessment and intervention do not hinge on negative stereotypes – assumptions need to be checked out. The common ethnocentric tendency of pathologizing black families, individuals or even whole communities is a very serious danger which must be avoided. For example, the ideological tendency to assume a higher level of criminality among black people (Marlow and Loveday, 2000) is a very destructive trap to fall into.

4   Following on from this is the need to help develop positive black identities. This applies particularly to areas such as fostering and adoption (Kirton, 2000), although this remains a contentious area. The issue of positive black identities is, however, a much wider one and would apply, for example, to social work with black elders (see Chapter 5). This is not to say that all black clients will need help in developing a positive identity, as that would be a reductionist oversimplification of a complex situation. It is none the less important to recognize the need to counter the potentially damaging effects of negative racist stereotypes (Robinson, 2008).

5   Affirmative action is, or should be, a fundamental basis of social work practice. This involves recognizing the accumulation of disadvantage black people have suffered as a result of racism and developing policies and practice which will help to overcome the difficulties this causes. Ignoring the need for affirmative action amounts to adopting a colourblind approach.

6   Combating racism is not simply a matter of purging one's own practice of discriminatory elements. It involves challenging racist comments, actions or attitudes in others and creating anti-racist alliances. From a collective position it is then possible to tackle racist structures and institutional practices in social work agencies and, to some extent at least, in other social welfare and related agencies. Setting out one's own anti-racist stall without seeking to influence others is a very narrow strategy with limited effectiveness.

7   In similar vein, it must be recognized that anti-discriminatory practice is the responsibility of not only practitioners, but also managers and educators. Managers have a role to play in setting an appropriate agenda,

supporting staff through the difficulties of establishing and maintaining anti-racist social work (Coulshed et al., 2006) and so on. Similarly, social work educators have a crucial role to play in laying the foundations for students to develop into skilled, knowledgeable and committed anti-discriminatory practitioners by helping workers and students to understand the nature of racist oppression and to begin to develop strategies for combating it. Practitioners, in turn, have a part to play in supporting and encouraging such work on the part of managers and educators and to offer constructive and supportive criticism where appropriate.

8   A strategy of 'permeation' is necessary. This means that issues of anti-racism should permeate policy, practice, management and training rather than be 'tagged on' as an additional consideration. Anti-racism should not be an optional extra but rather a fundamental dimension of our work. And this dimension needs to be linked to other important social divisions so that anti-racism is not seen in isolation from other efforts to promote equality and social justice and challenge oppression.

9   A central feature of anti-discriminatory practice in general and anti-racism in particular is that of empowerment. This involves seeking to help them to gain as much control as possible over their lives and circumstances. It is the opposite of creating dependency and subjecting clients to agency power (Thompson, 2007). As we have seen, social work with black and minority ethnic clients is characterized by an overemphasis on controlling at the expense of caring and supporting. Empowerment entails reversing that trend by using social work skills and resources in ways which support clients in overcoming racism.

10   The position of black workers employed in predominantly white organizations needs to be recognized. One common response has been the mistake of seeing anti-racism as the province mainly of black workers and assuming that, because someone is from an ethnic minority, they necessarily have the knowledge, skills and confidence to address racism. This can increase the sense of isolation and the pressure on black workers. Anti-racism must be a humanitarian endeavour in which black and white workers can work together to combat the oppression that black people – clients and colleagues – experience. Unless and until a supportive environment is created for black workers, the number of black social workers will remain low.

These ten points can, it is to be hoped, help people in social work to take their thinking and their practice forward towards an anti-racist social work. They cannot, of course, provide formula answers, but that is no bad thing. Moving away from formulas and stereotypes towards a more critical and informed approach is a basic tenet of anti-discriminatory practice (Thompson and Thompson, 2008).

Anti-racist social work is a complex area but this can be no excuse for failing to get to grips with the issues. As David Divine, one of the pioneers of anti-racist social work so aptly put it many years ago:

> There must be an obligation on us all to support and help each other in a climate conducive to honest and humble exchange. There are no 'right on' answers and approaches. Once we acknowledge that fact, further progress can be made.
>
> (Divine, 1990, p. 14)

Food for thought

- Consider your own ethnicity. How would you describe yourself?
- How might your ethnic or racial background be significant in delivering social work services?
- What racial stereotypes are you aware of? How can you ensure that these do not influence your practice?
- How can you find out more about the ethnic diversity of the communities you (will) work in?

Further resources

Again my own works are relevant (Thompson, 2007; 2011a; 2011b), but there is also a very significant worthwhile literature base that repays the time invested in drawing out the important lessons to be learned from it. Back and Solomos (*Theories of Race and Racism: A Reader*, 2009) provide a useful overview in the form of a set of readings. Solomos (*Race and Racism in Contemporary Britain*, 2003) and Pilkington (*Racial Disadvantage and Ethnic Diversity in Britain*, 2003) also provide good overviews of race and racism. Williams and Johnson (*Race and Ethnicity in a Welfare Society*, 2010) is an excellent discussion of the significance of race and ethnicity for welfare services. Kirton (*'Race', Ethnicity and Adoption*, 2000) tackles the thorny issue of adoption, while Alibhai-Brown (*Mixed Feelings: The Complex Lives of Mixed-Race Britons*, 2001) provides an interesting discussion of 'mixed race' Britons.

Garrett (2004) is an important book that rightly argues that anti-Irish racism should not be left out of the picture.

Robinson (*Psychology for Social Workers: Black Perspectives*, 2008) explores the changes needed to psychology to make it compatible with the needs and circumstances of black people, while Penketh (*Tackling Institutional Racism*, 2000) is a helpful analysis of institutional racism, as is Marlow and Loveday (*After Macpherson: Policing After the Stephen Lawrence Inquiry*, 2000). Farrell and Watt (*Responding to Racism in Ireland*, 2001) present discussions about racism in Ireland.

Malik (*Strange Fruit: Why Both Sides Are Wrong in the Race Debate*, 2008) is also a useful introduction to the complexities of this subject. Graham (*Social Work and African-Centred Worldviews*, 2002) is an important text which explores social work issues from an African-centred perspective. Other important works include: Jivraj and Simpson (*Ethnic Identity and Inequalities in Britain: The Dynamics of Diversity*, 2015); and Williams and Johnson (*Race and Ethnicity in a Welfare Society*, 2010).

CHAPTER 5

AGEISM AND ALIENATION

CHAPTER OVERVIEW

In this chapter you will:

- Begin to understand how age serves as a basis for discrimination; the chapter focuses on older people but there are also significant implications in relation to discrimination against children and young people
- Appreciate how common ageism is and how harmful it can be
- Explore strategies for avoiding and challenging ageism in professional practice

Introduction

The terms 'sexism' and 'racism' have long been established in the English language and are not seen as technical terms or jargon. The term 'ageism', however, is much less well established and, although being used more and more in social work and related disciplines, it has only recently begun to enter the vocabulary of everyday speech. This would seem to be a reflection of the lack of awareness of ageism and the questions it raises, and also an indication of its relatively low status as an area of study. This very fact is itself characteristic of ageism – the marginalization of issues relating to age, particularly the problems of old age.

Age is a social division; it is a dimension of the social structure on the basis of which power, privilege and opportunities tend to be allocated. Age is not just a simple matter of biological maturation – it is a highly significant social indicator. This is the case whatever our age – all ages are imbued with social significance – but as we shall see, old age has special consequences in terms of the attachment of meaning to life stages. The focus in this chapter is therefore on the social position of older people and what implications this has for social work with this client group, although much of what is discussed here is also relevant to work with children and young people, as they too can experience ageism – discrimination on the grounds of age (see S. Thompson, 2005).

For a variety of reasons, including the effects of demographic changes now being felt, social work with older people is attracting far more attention than has ever been the case in the past. It is important, then, that due regard is given to questions of good practice in working with older people – that is, to the development of anti-ageist practice.

When we consider that social work with older people has considerable discriminatory potential, there is a serious danger that overworked staff will inadvertently increase the degree of oppression experienced by older people. This situation adds even greater weight to the argument that a clear understanding of ageism and the foundations of anti-ageist practice should be a high priority for workers in this field. This chapter attempts to begin that process of understanding.

What is ageism?

In what has now become a classic definition, Hughes and Mtezuka described ageism as: 'the social process through which negative images of and attitudes towards older people, based solely on the characteristics of old age itself, result in discrimination' (1992, p. 220). The concept of ageism dates back to the 1960s and the work of Butler (Phillipson, 2000). Butler offered a definition of the term in which the three levels or dimensions of **P**, **C** and **S** are reflected:

> Ageism makes it easier to ignore the frequently poor social and economic plight of older people. We can avoid dealing with the reality that our productivity-minded society has little use for non-producers – in this case those who have reached an arbitrarily defined retirement age ... Ageism is manifested in a wide range of phenomena, both on individual and institutional levels – stereotypes and myths, outright disdain and dislike, or simply subtle avoidance of contact; discriminatory practices in housing, employment and services of all kinds; epithets, cartoons and jokes.
>
> (Butler, 1975, p. 12)

Butler recognizes the personal and institutional levels and relates the latter to structural issues such as productivity and, until recently, the state-defined retirement age. The cultural level manifests itself in 'epithets, cartoons and jokes', as older people are frequently the objects of cruel humour – a reflection of their low status and the lack of respect accorded to them by dominant cultural values.

I shall focus later in this chapter on the structural dimension by considering the political economy approach of theorists such as Chris Phillipson. But for now the emphasis will be on the personal and cultural levels. In particular, I shall explore a number of common assumptions which both reflect and reinforce ageism. I shall expound each of these assumptions or 'equations' in turn:

Old equals useless   This is the 'burden' model of old age. Older people are seen as 'past their best', no longer productive, no longer contributing to the economy and therefore a burden, a drain on the state's resources (Powell, 2006). This is often used as an excuse for not providing a service or for giving preferential treatment to younger people.

Old equals childlike   Old age is often seen as a period of 'postadulthood' (Midwinter, 1990), as if having returned to a second childhood. Older people can find they are having decisions made for them (for example, by professionals or relatives) without consultation or their rights are being overlooked or they are being patronized, for example, in the way they are referred to ('the old dear'). These are examples of what Hockey and James (1993) termed 'infantilization', a process parallel to the demeaning tendency to refer to adult women as 'girls'.

Old equals not like children   Paradoxically, older people are not treated like children in terms of an equivalent level of protection or provision of services. Social work with older people is often marginalized and treated as the 'poor relation' compared with more prestigious forms of practice, such as child care (Thompson, 2002c).

Old equals ill   As a general rule, it is true that the greater one's age, the higher the incidence of illness will be. However, this is a long way from the commonly held assumption that all or even most older people are ill. Some people even think of old age as an illness. But, in reality, the extent of illness and infirmity in old age is grossly exaggerated and misunderstood (Bond and Cabrero, 2007).

Old equals not ill   Once again we have a paradox. When older people are genuinely ill (that is, they are not simply the victims of an ageist assumption), they often meet resistance and their symptoms can easily be dismissed with a comment such as: 'What do you expect at your age?' This is reflected in health service priorities as, for example, when old age is seen as a contraindication for some forms of treatment (Sidell, 1995).

Old equals lonely   Older people are often subjected to considerable pity as they are deemed to be 'lonely'. No doubt many older people are lonely, as indeed are many younger people. However, very many elderly people have a good social network and are not lonely (Victor, Scambler and Bond, 2009). In addition, it is a mistake to equate being alone with being lonely. Whether someone is lonely or not needs to be assessed. Someone who lives alone may have a high level of what has come to be known as 'social capital' (Lin, 2002) – that is, personal relationships, group associations and other social contacts that enrich their life. To assume that an older person is lonely, without actually checking, is an ageist assumption.

Old equals asexual   Sexuality in children tends to be discouraged and is seen as something 'reserved for adults'. However, following on from the second point above, it is significant that sexual activity among older people is often frowned upon or even seen as 'disgusting'. For example, an older man with a strong libido is described derogatively as a 'dirty old man' (de Beauvoir, 1977, p. 53) whereas his younger counterpart attracts more socially acceptable, albeit sexist, terms such as 'young buck'. Older people are thus denied their sexuality (Gott and Hinchliff, 2003).

Voice of experience 5.1

It has always struck me as odd that a natural phenomenon like sexuality is seen as something to laugh at or to regard it as strange or somehow not right. It's as if there is an unwritten rule that when you get to a certain age it is wrong to have sexual feelings or to want intimacy. *Siobhan, a social worker in a re-ablement team*

Old equals unintelligent   Older people are often perceived as being less intelligent than younger people. There is often an implicit assumption that intellectual capacities are lower, if not significantly lower, for those people who have reached old age. This can be accompanied by an assumption that confusion is a 'normal' part of the ageing process. Thus older people are expected to be slow on the uptake and unable to understand complex issues. This, in turn, can lead to workers talking to them in an oversimplified, thus patronizing way.

Old equals poor   It has long been recognized that class differences tend to be magnified in old age, and so poorer people may suffer considerable poverty when they reach old age (Cann and Dean, 2009). However, important though this is, we should not allow it to persuade us that old people, as a social group, are poor. Very many indeed are, but to begin one's assessment of an older person with the assumption that he or she is poor can lead to considerable problems and could involve overlooking available solutions to presenting problems.

Old equals less than human   There is a strong ideological tendency to dismiss older people, to deny them their humanity. I found a good example of this in an article in a newsletter of a local 'Alcohol Forum'. The author, a psychiatrist, is discussing safe limits for weekly alcohol consumption when he comments that: 'Safety limits are proposed in terms of alcohol units per week (10) but these limits are for males or females, not for the elderly'. Although the good intentions of the author are apparent elsewhere in the article, the common tendency to distinguish between 'ordinary people' (that is, males and females) and 'the elderly' is clearly in evidence.

This is not an exhaustive list and much more could be said on the topic. However, having gone some way towards clarifying what ageism is and what form it takes, let us now turn our attention to how these issues apply to social work.

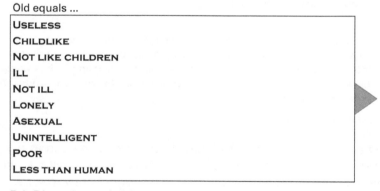

Old equals ...

USELESS
CHILDLIKE
NOT LIKE CHILDREN
ILL
NOT ILL
LONELY
ASEXUAL
UNINTELLIGENT
POOR
LESS THAN HUMAN

Figure 5.1 Distortions of old age

The implications for social work

One manifestation of institutional ageism is the tendency for social work with older people to be seen as routine and uninteresting and more suited to unqualified workers and social work assistants than to qualified social workers. Indeed, some people argue, for this reason, that care management is not social work – see Thompson and Thompson (2005), for a view which strongly challenges this. For many staff, work with older people is seen as primarily matching service to need – a far cry from the problem solving and empowerment ethos of social work (Thompson 2009a). It is relatively easy mistake to make to focus on service provision without considering skills and methods of intervention (Thompson and Thompson, 2005).

Practice focus 5.1

Chandra was a social worker in a mental health team. He worked with people from different age groups. However, he gradually came to specialize in working with older people. As he did so, he began to adapt more and more of his mental health knowledge, skills and methods of working to this older client group. He saw the development of this knowledge and skill base as particularly important, as he was aware of the danger of reducing work with older people to low levels of routine practice.

Ageism has two sets of implications for social work assessment. The first relates to the points raised above. That is, assessment needs to address not only simple notions of need and service availability, but also wider issues which form part of a comprehensive assessment. The second relates directly to ageism and can be subdivided into two parts. On the one hand, assessment should include consideration of the impact of ageism on older people's lives, including, as we shall see below, low self-esteem, feelings of being a nuisance and so on. On the other hand, care needs to be taken to ensure that ageist assumptions are not influencing the assessment work being undertaken. As with racism and sexism, if we are not actively 'swimming against the tide' of cultural and structural ageism, we will be carried along with it, such is the strength of ageist ideology.

In similar vein, Jack describes older people as being among the most disempowered of our citizens:

Disempowered, that is, by poverty, poor housing and inadequate and frequently discriminatory health and social services. It is particularly important at this time to recognize the need for empowerment among older people because the so-called 'elderly' – a diverse population of ten million people between 60 and 100 plus – are increasingly being identified by cost-conscious governments, local authorities and service providers as a 'problem' due to their increasing numbers and, allegedly, greater consumption of health and social services. This constitutes a very real threat to those arbitrarily assigned to this 'group' and all those claiming an interest in empowerment will therefore be concerned particularly with the plight of elderly people.

(Jack, 1995a, p. 7)

These issues can therefore be seen as major factors that can affect our assessment of situations, in the sense that we may add to the disempowerment or contribute more positively to empowerment, depending on how aware we are of the operation of ageist processes and how prepared we are for dealing with them. Ageism therefore has major implications for assessment, and our awareness of ageism should flag up a number of dangers for us, such as assessment becoming nothing more than a test of eligibility for service (Milner and O'Byrne, 2009). Similarly, it is important that assessment should not be simply part of a brokerage role within the context of care management:

Assessment is a process closely associated with care management and community care. However, it is important to note that it can also be used in a much broader sense. For example, the first stage in any problem-solving process is likely to be an assessment – a gathering of information and the development of an action plan ... It extends far beyond the assessment of needs implicit in care management.

This is an important point to make, as assessment is a process that all staff working with older people are likely to be involved with at one time or another.

(Thompson, 1995a, p. 81)

To ignore the significance of assessment in working with older people can therefore be seen as an example of ageism in its own right.

But ageism also applies to other aspects of social work. One major aspect of this is the danger of what Sue Thompson (2005) calls 'welfarism', the tendency to focus on the 'needs' of older people in welfare terms, to pay scant attention to their strengths and, in so doing, exaggerate the extent of the problems experienced in old age (see also Powell, 2006). This is applicable at two levels. In general terms, there is an often unspoken (**C** level) assumption that being old entails being in need of welfare services – but this needs to be balanced against the fact that only a relatively small proportion of people over retirement age receive social services assistance.

More specifically, in relation to those older people who do become service users, welfarism can easily present them as a 'series of problems', rather than real people who have not only problems and needs but also strengths, assets and a positive contribution to make (S. Thompson, 2009).

Key point 5.1

It is ironic that discrimination can often arise from a caring attitude. That is, people who are not tuned in to the subtleties of discrimination may find that their efforts to be helpful and supportive have unintentional discriminatory consequences.

One implication of this is that oppressive ageist practices can actually be perpetuated by the good intentions of workers and general public alike, who see a 'welfarist' approach to older people as kind and humane. The influence of ageist ideology ensures that the demeaning and patronizing nature of welfarism is rarely realized by those who hold such views. As with anti-racism, good intentions alone are not enough. Indeed, welfarism shows that unenlightened good intentions can unwittingly reflect and reinforce ageist stereotypes.

Taking these issues a step further, the emphasis on care rather than empowerment can lead to health and social care staff increasing the dependency of the elderly people in their care (Thompson and Thompson, 2001). The word 'dependency' is an important one, as it is instrumental in creating a negative image of older people and gives credence to notions of older people as a nuisance or a burden. It is therefore vitally important that social work staff do not use the term loosely or uncritically.

Dependency and the associated term of frailty imply a medical model, one which focuses on physical capabilities and their decline or dysfunction. Such an approach runs the risk of oversimplifying the complex range of factors surrounding old age and reducing these to a medical or biological level. A helpful concept in this regard is 'interdependence', which Wilson links to the equally important concept of 'reciprocity' (the ability to be able to give as well as receive and the importance for self-esteem and well-being of being able to do so):

> As long as older men and women can fulfil the norms of reciprocity they can see themselves as more or less independent but, if they feel they have nothing to offer in return for support, they are likely to feel disempowered and a burden. They are also more likely to be described as a burden by

those who finance or care for them. ... [This] model sees interdependence as an essential part of being human and takes it for granted as a 'natural' aspect of family and community relations.

(Wilson, 2000, p. 116)

The optimism inherent in this conception of how older people can be seen as *inter*dependent where they are not denied opportunities for reciprocity (S. Thompson, 2009) is certainly to be welcomed, especially in the context of a social work with older people which is often dismissed as routine and uninteresting or reserved for unqualified staff. Social work with older people is seen as less prestigious than, say, childcare, and this in itself is a reflection of ageism, based on the negative assumption that practice with older people requires fewer skills and less application.

Ageism also manifests itself in terms of the social policy context and legislative framework. For example, it has long been recognized that older people's needs are covered by the same legislative and policy umbrella as disabled or infirm people, thus indicating that such people are considered a sufficiently homogeneous group to be catered for in this way – despite their varying needs and circumstances. Policy in relation to community care can also be seen to follow this pattern and reveal an assumption that there is no need for a clear policy in relation to older people, as it is presumed that they can be 'tagged on' to other policies.

There is also a further dimension of the policy context in terms of older people and decision making. Making decisions for children without consulting them may be considered by many as poor parenting, and would certainly be seen as poor social work practice. In the case of older people, however, such an infringement of civil liberties is not uncommon. As Tanner comments: 'rendering audible the voices of those who are seldom heard can be seen in itself as a route to empowerment' (2010, p. 24). This denial of citizenship can be linked directly to ageism and, more specifically, to the notion of 'infantilization' – the tendency to treat older people as if they were children (Hockey and James, 1993). Social workers therefore need to be wary of colluding with this by falling into the trap of listening to the carer(s) without hearing the voice of the older person. As Sue Thompson rightly argues:

An anti-ageist approach requires us to work in partnership with the people concerned, and it is difficult to see how this can be done without listening. This is not necessarily easy in every circumstance, but that does not mean that this important principle should be abandoned. ... Listening is always important in people work of any type as if forms a basis on which partnership working can flourish. It is perhaps particularly so when working with those whose wishes and life chances are so often compromised by ageist assumptions and preconceptions.

(S. Thompson, 2005, p. 40)

Ageism entails devaluing and marginalizing older people, dismissing their contribution and their needs and presenting them as a burden or nuisance. The ageism inherent in social and economic policy leaves many older people and their carers as a low priority in terms of service provision. All this combines to give rise to a number of situations in which the stresses and tensions are increasingly likely to lead to abuse. Ageism is therefore a significant factor.

A further implication of ageism for social work is the way the oppression experienced by older people can be internalized and manifest itself as low self-esteem. As is the case with racism and sexism, the stereotypical assumptions and expectations associated with ageism can be internalized by older people. Indeed, it is not surprising that a group of people who are constantly receiving strong negative messages should perceive themselves in strongly negative terms. This can have the effect of lowering morale and sapping confidence.

High self-esteem is premised on receiving positive messages, feeling valued and important but, as we have seen, ageism acts as a significant barrier to receiving such positive signals. Social work staff need to be sensitive to these issues in order to:

(a) avoid reinforcing negative and demeaning images; and

(b) seek opportunities to give positive feedback and enhance self-esteem.

A major component of successfully achieving high self-esteem is that of maintaining a thread of meaning to one's life – having targets to aim for and goals to achieve. As Simone de Beauvoir puts it: 'There is only one solution if old age is not to be an absurd parody of our former life, and that is to go on pursuing ends that give our existence a meaning' (de Beauvoir, 1977, p. 601). She then goes on to give examples of some possibilities: 'devotion to individuals, to groups or to causes, social, political, intellectual or creative work' (ibid.). She argues that our lives have value if we attribute value to the lives of others – through love, friendship, compassion or even indignation (see also S. Thompson, 2009, for a discussion of how the important notion of reciprocity – giving as well as receiving – fits in well with this picture).

These are important lessons for social workers and social care workers. Ageism would have us focus on 'care' and dependency. Anti-ageist practice would have us look to purposeful activity, meaning, value and esteem.

The task is not just to 'look after', but also to motivate, empower and promote self-esteem (Thompson and Thompson, 2001).

Closely related to the notion of self-esteem is that of dignity. Dignity refers to the intrinsic worth of human beings and is therefore an important word in the anti-ageist vocabulary (SCIE, 2006). Set against this is the concept of 'risk', or more specifically protection from risk. In a classic work, Norman (1980) discusses a number of ways in which dignity and self-determination can be sacrificed in the name of protection from risk. In a later article she argues that 'an honest approach to the management of risk' should be part of a strategy in which improved professional practice can address issues of ageism (Norman, 1987, p. 14).

Referring to the work of Brearley (1982), she comments on the need to understand risk as a matter of 'gambling', by weighing the dangers inherent in a particular situation against the potential benefits. She then goes on to clarify this by giving a concrete example:

> Does the physical safety of the move to live with a caring daughter or to residential care outweigh the psychological dangers of loss of independence? Does the danger to a daughter's health, earning power and family relationships outweigh the guilt and stress she feels in the present situation?
>
> (Norman, 1987, p. 15)

The balance of risk is an important aspect of social work with older people and, from the perspective of anti-discriminatory practice, we must be wary of allowing ageist ideology to tilt the balance in favour of an over-cautious, perhaps somewhat paternalistic, approach.

Practice focus 5.2

Mrs Linton lived alone and had no relatives in the area. Her neighbour, Mrs Jarvis, was becoming increasingly concerned about her and often contacted Social Services, the GP and the health visitor. However, Mrs Linton remained adamant that she did not need anyone's help and refused to receive services of any kind. At first, Mrs Jarvis felt that Mrs Linton should be forced to receive help for her own good. Eventually she came to accept that her elderly neighbour had the right to refuse services and, like many older people, chose to exercise that right. (Thompson, 1995a, p. 48)

Ageism manifests itself at all three levels – personal, cultural and structural – and so the implications for social work staff reach far and wide. The development of anti-ageist practice therefore presents a major challenge for all concerned. I shall outline some of the steps towards anti-ageist practice later in this chapter by way of conclusion. First, however, it is necessary to examine some of the arguments which have arisen in response to ageist ideology.

The anti-ageist response

In a text that became a foundation stone of the 'political economy' approach to old age, Phillipson makes the important point that: 'undue weight has been given to biological and psychological changes in old age (and the deterioration seen to accompany them), in contrast to the role played by the economic and political environment' (1982, p. 2). He links negative attitudes towards older people to the structural requirements of the capitalist quest for profit. He argues that old age is seen as 'non-productive' and 'a period of social redundancy' (ibid., p. 7). But this is no coincidence – this negative and dismissive ideology is pervasive because it is linked inextricably with the economic requirements of the capitalist system.

Older people are seen as marginal to the labour market and are therefore assigned a lower status due to the emphasis on measuring social value in terms of one's contribution to the production of wealth. Old age therefore needs to be understood in economic and political terms. This approach has proven to be an influential approach which has tended to counterbalance the traditional perspective on old age which sees this life stage as predominantly a medical problem as if old age were primarily a disease process (Powell, 2006). Indeed, as noted in Chapter 1, 'medicalization' can be seen as an aspect of ageism, part of the social construction of old age as a problem.

Theorists who adopt a structural approach to old age are therefore keen to emphasize the social, political and economic influences on the situation of older people. That is, they see old age as a period of 'structured dependency' which is socially constructed rather than biologically determined.

Voice of experience 5.2

When I took over as manager I was concerned that there was a strong medical feel to the place, with a strong emphasis on looking after people who were – as my ex-boss used to put it – 'ailing and failing'. Staff seemed to take the idea of dependency as the norm. I had to work hard to get them to recognize the problems involved in that sort of negative approach. Of course, we had to recognize people's needs and difficulties, but we also had to focus on strengths and positives. People working in child care often talk about resilience in children, but it's an important factor for older people too, of course. *Jenny, a day services manager*

The work of Bytheway and Johnson was also important in developing an understanding of how ageism manifests itself in a biological interpretation of the ageing process: 'Ageism is a set of beliefs originating in the biological variations between people and relating to the ageing process' (1990, p. 36). They then go on to present what they see as four central pillars of an anti-ageist response:

1 *Abandon ageist language*   We should avoid grouping people together according to their age. Age should be referred to only when necessary. (See also Chapter 2 for a discussion of ageist language.)

2 *Recognize age for what it is*   What is required is an assertion of personhood, a continuing personal sense of social identity and a popular acceptance of the realities of ageing. If it is argued, for example, that life is a continuing process of development and 'becoming', then this implies that age does matter and is valued (p. 137).

3 *Avoid the restrictions of chronological age*   How old a person is should not be used as a stipulation (for example, in determining eligibility for a service). Individuals or groups should not be excluded from jobs, services, participation and so on purely on the grounds of age.

4 *Abandon the 'us–them' mentality*   We are all subject to the ageing process. We should be aware of this and therefore avoid separating off 'the old': 'the most damaging thing we can do – contributing immensely to the power of ageism – is to seemingly deny that "we" who discuss these issues are somehow freed of the reality of the ageing experience' (p. 38).

In the same year that this article was published, the Church of England also added its weight to the development of anti-ageism. A report from the Board for Social Responsibility, entitled simply 'Ageing', drew attention to the: 'negative attitudes to ageing that are widespread in industrialized societies' (1990, p. 140).

The report linked ageism to two major factors and these were:

● fear of death; and

● a materialistic culture which equates success with productivity and economic activity.

It is these issues, the report contended, which lead to stereotypical negative attitudes towards older people and an undervaluing of their positive contribution to society. The report went on to argue that the Church could play a more positive role in tackling ageism both within its own institutional structures and practices and in wider society as a whole. Two decades later the report's analysis and recommendations continue to apply.

The role of the fear of death is one which also features in the work of de Beauvoir. In particular she questions the notion of death being near for older people:

> The old man knows that he will die soon; the fatality is as present at seventy as it is at eighty, and the word 'soon' remains as vague at eighty as it did at seventy. It is not correct to speak of a relationship with death: the fact is that the old man, like other men, has a relationship with life and nothing else.
>
> (de Beauvoir, 1977, p. 492)

In short, old age has more to do with life than it has to do with death. And this 'affirmation' of life is a key part of the existentialist philosophy on which de Beauvoir's work is based. But it is perhaps the other strand of her thinking, her seminal role in the development of feminism, which should interest us more here. For what we need to recognize is that ageism does not operate in isolation. It intersects with other forms of discrimination, such as sexism and racism. These combinations of oppression are significant for social work practice, and so they are worthy of closer attention. A discussion of these areas forms the subject matter of the following section.

Multiple oppressions

For demographic reasons the world of older people is predominantly a female world, as women far outnumber men in the later stages of life. The interrelationship of old age and gender therefore takes on a particular significance (Arber, Davidson and Ginn, 2003). It is not simply a mathematical matter of adding sexism to ageism. The reality is much more complex than this. Older women will have a long and cumulative experience of sexism and will also have lived through a period of considerable change as far as social attitudes to women are concerned. The impact of sexism on older women and the effects of the interaction of sexism and ageism cannot therefore be routinely or straightforwardly predicted. These are empirical, rather than theoretical, matters – that is, they cannot be determined in advance; they need to be examined. There are, however, broad principles and characteristics which can be discerned. For example, there are significant issues in relation to self-esteem. Maintaining a degree of dignity and self-worth can be seen to be more difficult for older women due to the structural and ideological constraints, and this, in turn, can lead to a sense of 'postadulthood' and infantilization, as discussed earlier in this chapter (but see Arber, Davidson and Ginn, 2003, for a discussion of the advantages women can have over men in old age).

Both these aspects, gender and age, also intersect with issues of race and ethnicity (Walker, 2009). The Report of the Board for Social Responsibility discussed earlier also argued that:

> The special needs of elderly members of minority ethnic groups will become more important over the next few decades as the population ages and its profile becomes similar to that of the white population. One implication for policy making is the urgency of making sure that health and welfare services are sensitive to the needs of these groups.
>
> (Board for Social Responsibility, 1990, p. 18)

And this sensitivity will also need to apply to the dimension of gender. Age, gender and race/ethnicity are fundamental aspects of our experience, and social work and social care practice need to be based on at least a basic understanding of these issues and how they interact in specific cases and particular contexts (see *Promoting Equality*, 2011a).

And, as if this were not complex enough, we must also take account of the socioeconomic dimension – that of class. As has been noted, class differences in early life tend to be amplified in old age, thus accounting in part for the higher incidence of poverty among older people (Scharf, 2009).

The marginalization resulting from low income is reinforced and extended by the additional discriminatory impact of both racism and ageism.

This combination of sources of discrimination is an important element in the social context of ethnic minority elders. It therefore needs to feature in social work assessments and interventions and, on a wider scale, policies and service plans. Oppression is both a social injustice and a barrier to self-realization and, as such, the removal, reduction and prevention of oppression are valid and legitimate aims for social work. Where two or more such oppressions combine or intersect, their impact can be even more significant, the resulting disempowerment even more far reaching.

Practice focus 5.3

Jackie was a care manager in a large urban authority, having recently moved from a rural area some distance away. She was finding it difficult to adjust to her new environment but was coping quite well. However, one case she was asked to deal with was quite unlike anything she had previously encountered. Mrs Singh was an 82-year-old woman whose origins lay in India. Since coming to Britain in the early 1950s she had lived in very poor housing with very limited income, in addition to which she had experienced racist taunts and abuse and physical violence at the hands of her late husband. Jackie felt quite over-whelmed by the sheer intensity of oppression Mrs Singh had encountered and for a little while she felt paralysed by it all, unable to respond. When she was able to respond and began to come to terms with the situation, she realized just how important it was to understand, and counter, the effects of discrimination in people's lives.

The point that this discussion reinforces is the need to adopt a holistic framework, an anti-discriminatory perspective which takes account of not only racism or sexism but also ageism and disablism (and indeed the other forms of discrimination that characterize our society). But this holistic framework must be applicable to actual practice if it is to be of value. The final section of this chapter therefore addresses some of the key issues involved in drawing on such anti-discriminatory theory in practice.

Towards anti-ageist practice

Social work with older people has often been seen as low priority, relatively routine and undemanding work, although this view, in itself, is a reflection of ageist ideology and reveals a rather conde-scending (and misguided) attitude towards this area of work.

> ### Key point 5.2
>
> Sadly many people pay a high level of attention to such well-documented forms of discrimination as racism and sexism while largely ignoring other significant sources of oppression, such as ageism. A genuinely anti-discriminatory practice must be prepared to recognize and counter all forms of unfair discrimination, not just those that have received the most attention.

It is important to be clear about what the social work task entails and how it can be achieved within the context of anti-discriminatory practice. It is therefore necessary to consider the steps required to move towards an anti-ageist practice. Some of these are outlined here.

1   Ageist stereotypes can easily seduce us into making negative assumptions about older people and thus establishing a framework for discrimination and oppression. Anti-ageist practice is therefore premised on avoiding and challenging ageist assumptions and myths. This is particularly important in relation to the process of assessment. In fact, if we are not vigilant, assumptions can masquerade as assessment. The maxim should therefore be: *assess, don't assume!*

2   Much of the literature in relation to old age is from a medical perspective; old age is often presented as if it were a disease or pathological state. This has significant implications in terms of the construction of role expectations and attitudes. This, in turn, can have a major impact on self-image and thus on self-esteem. The ageism inherent in a medicalized approach to older people is a pitfall which social work must avoid. A key part of this is to cease using medical terminology in a social work context – for example, to speak of assessment and intervention, rather than diagnosis and treatment.

3   Traditional social work is partly geared towards helping people 'adjust' to their personal and social circumstances. The problem with this is that it is a reductionist approach, in so far as it reduces a complex psychosocial situation to a straightforward matter of pathology or individual failing. Anti-ageist practice needs to transcend notions of 'adjustment' and focus instead on empowerment – the development of older people's personal power and seeking ways of increasing their control over their lives and circumstances (for example, through advocacy or access to resources).

4 Townsend (2007) discusses social policy's role in producing, or at least, reinforcing what can be described as 'structured dependency'. Social welfare practice can play a part in constructing or increasing dependency in older people. It is therefore essential, in moving towards anti-ageist practice, for social work to be active in avoiding dependency-creation. We should aim for 'interdependency' – the mutuality and human affirmation involved in helping each other.

5 Ageism marginalizes older people and casts them in secondary roles or presents them as useless and a burden to society. In view of this, we should not be surprised if many older people struggle to maintain a thread of meaning or sense of purpose to their lives and thus fall prey to low spirits or depression. In countering this, V. W. Marshall's notion of 'authorship' should be a useful part of the anti-ageist social worker's repertoire. It is a concept akin to empowerment – having a sense of being in control of one's life, and, as Marshall stresses, of one's death: 'if people want their lives to be meaningful stories with good endings, they also want to be the authors. This is the taking of responsibility for one's life as a whole, including its ending in death' (1986a, p. 142). Social work staff must not shy away from issues of death or dying for these are part of life, of meaning and of personal responsibility (Thompson and Thompson, 2016).

6 Ageism, as with other forms of oppression and discrimination, is both reflected in, and constructed by, language. Anti-ageist social work therefore needs to be sensitive to the role of language and thus avoid ageist and depersonalizing terms such as 'the elderly'. We should always remember to add the word 'people', that is, 'elderly people', or better still 'older people'. The term 'elders' is also a positively valued one, especially as it has connotations of respect and dignity. Social work staff often use demeaning and perhaps patronizing terms to refer to their older clients, but may be doing so in good faith without realizing their negative impact. Examples of this would be: 'old dears', 'my old darlings' and so on. What is needed, therefore, is a greater sensitivity to language, so that it can become a tool of anti-ageism rather than a sign of unchallenged ageism.

7 The effectiveness and appropriateness of help offered and work undertaken will depend in large part on the quality of the assessment which establishes the framework for intervention. It is therefore important that such assessment should be holistic – taking account of a wide range of factors. The trap which lures many an unsuspecting worker is the routine matching of service to need.

This is an 'off the peg' approach in which the complex process of assessment is reduced to checking eligibility for services available (Thompson and Thompson, 2005; Thompson, 2009a). This latter approach is too narrow and restrictive in its scope and has no impact on service development. It has no place in a genuinely anti-ageist practice.

8 Ageism has the effect of undermining a sense of dignity and the self-esteem which partly depends on it. Ageism marginalizes, excludes and demoralizes. A key task within a programme of developing anti-ageist practice must therefore be the promotion of dignity and the enhancement of self-esteem – a counterbalance to the prevalence of negative stereotypes. In effect, this is not a single task, but rather an aspect of all the tasks undertaken in work with older people – an essential dimension or underlying principle of all our dealings with older people.

9 One significant aspect of ageist ideology is the process of infantilization – treating older people as if they were children. This manifests itself in relation to the question of taking risks. Social work has followed the medical profession in adopting a rather protective approach to this issue. As Norman (1987) puts it: 'we deny them, as we deny children, the right to take responsibility for their sexuality, their behaviour and their risk-taking' (1987, p. 14). In recognizing this we must also recognize that the more protective we become the more we challenge older people's rights to make their own decisions and be responsible for themselves. Anti-ageist practice needs to ensure that the protection offered is not at the expense of rights.

10 Anti-ageism is not a separate area of practice. It needs to be seen in relation to sexism and racism and, indeed other forms of discrimination that may affect older people. These are fundamental aspects of human experience and need to be understood in relation to each other. Anti-ageism needs to be part of the wider enterprise and challenge of anti-discriminatory practice. The lessons learned from anti-racism and anti-sexism must also be applied to anti-ageism. They are not in conflict or competition but, rather, part of the wider movement towards an emancipatory social work.

These are all important steps towards putting anti-ageism firmly on the social work agenda and, moreover, making it a reality in day-to-day practice.

Food for thought

● Consider your current age. What advantages and disadvantages does your age bestow upon you at the moment, given society's attitudes towards different people at different stages in the life course?

● What stereotypes of older people are you aware of? How can you ensure that these are not allowed to influence your practice?

● In what ways are older people treated like children and in what way are they not?

● If you work with children and young people, which points made in this chapter also apply to them?

Further resources

Sue Thompson's short text is an ideal introduction (*Age Discrimination*, 2005). Powell (*Social Theory and Aging*, 2006), Tanner (*Managing the Ageing Experience: Learning from Older People*, 2010) and Nolan, Davies and Grant (*Working with Older People: Key Issues in Policy and Practice*, 2001) also offer some useful insights, while Cann and Dean (*Unequal Ageing: The Untold Story of Exclusion in Old Age*, 2009) are particularly strong on inequality issues.

Sue Thompson (*From Where I'm Sitting*, 2002a) is very relevant to those working with older people in residential, day care and home care settings. Its main strength is that it addresses the issues from the point of view of the older person. Sue Thompson ('Old Age', 2002b) addresses issues of loss and grief in old age, as does Thompson and Thompson ('Older People', 2004).

Arber, Davidson and Ginn (2003) provide important insights into gender and ageing. There are several good collections of readings on working with older people: Bernard and Scharf (*Critical Perspectives on Ageing Societies*, 2009); Bond et al. (*Ageing in Society: European Perspectives on Gerontology*, 2007); and Gilleard and Higgs (*Contexts of Ageing: Class, Cohort and Community*, 2005). Hornstein (*Outlawing Age Discrimination: Foreign Lessons, UK Choices*, 2001) provides an international perspective on age discrimination, as does Timonen (*Ageing Societies: A Comparative Introduction*, 2008).

Phillipson (*Capitalism and the Construction of Old Age*, 1982) and Fennell, Phillipson and Evers (*The Sociology of Old Age*, 1988) are now both a little dated, but are classic texts that are well worth consulting.

Thompson and Thompson ('Empowering Older People: Beyond the Care Model', 2001) discuss moving away from traditional approaches to working with older people towards a model based on empowerment. Cattan (*Mental Health and*

Well-Being in Later Life, 2009) provides an informative discussion about mental health and well-being in later life.

Multiple experiences of discrimination are discussed in Simpson (*Middle-Aged men, Ageing and Ageism: Over the Rainbow?*, 2015) and Sargeant (*Age Discrimination and Diversity: Multiple Discrimination from An Age Perspective*, 2011).

Other important texts include: Edmondson and von Kondratowitz (*Valuing Older People*, 2009) and Powell and Chamberlain (*Social Welfare, Aging and Social Theory*, 2012).

CHAPTER 6

DISABILITY AND SOCIAL HANDICAP

CHAPTER OVERVIEW

In this chapter you will:

- Learn about how disability is a major basis of (often unwitting) discrimination
- Recognize that such discrimination is rooted in widespread social attitudes towards disability and is not simply a matter of the prejudice of a bigoted minority
- Explore the implications of disablism for professional practice

Introduction

The field of social work with disabled people is a long-established one but it is only since the development of the Disabled People's Movement that the basis of this work has been seriously questioned and challenged. The old assumptions and certainties are no longer intact and a very different approach to issues of disability is now firmly on the agenda.

The development of the Disabled People's Movement introduced a new, politicized approach to meeting the needs of disabled people, an approach which is highly critical of traditional perspectives on this area of social work practice. This approach is based on a social – rather than medical or psychological – model of disability and, as we shall see in more detail below, this entails quite a significant shift in how disability is to be perceived, understood and acted upon.

Social work with disabled people has never achieved a priority status and has, to a large extent, been marginalized as a minority special interest, often receiving minimal attention on professional qualifying courses. It has also often been subsumed within medical discourse and seen as a paramedical undertaking somewhat distanced from mainstream social work (parallel with health-related social work). It is thus given low status, low levels of funding and relatively little attention in terms of research and professional development.

This state of affairs can itself be seen as discriminatory and indicative of the marginalized and negatively valued position of disabled people and issues concerned with their well-being. This is illustrative of what has become known as disablism, systematic discrimination against people with disabilities which produces a milieu of oppression and degradation.

What is disablism?

Disablism is a relatively new concept to be introduced into social work theory and practice. Like ageism, however, it is steadily gaining ground and achieving greater currency. This is important, as the issues cannot be confronted and problems resolved until they are firmly on the agenda. And to do this we need the vocabulary; we need to name the enemy we are fighting in order to recognize it and muster our resources against it.

Disablism is therefore an important term, even if the introduction of another 'ism' does seem trite and could lead some less sensitive people to dismiss it as an academic fad. Disablism refers to the combination of social forces, cultural values and personal prejudices which marginalizes disabled people, portrays them in a negative light and thus oppresses them. This combination encapsulates a powerful ideology which has the effect of denying disabled people full participation in mainstream social life. As Oliver comments:

> The barriers disabled people encounter include inaccessible education systems, working environments, inadequate disability benefits, discriminatory health and social support services, inaccessible transport, houses and public buildings and amenities, and the devaluing of disabled people through negative images in the media films, television and newspapers.
>
> (Oliver, 2009, p. 47)

Such barriers are ideological as well as physical. Disablism therefore incorporates an undermining of citizenship, a point to which I shall return in more detail below.

Disablism shares many of the features of ageism: a tendency towards infantilization, a patronizing 'does she take sugar?' attitude, an assumption of illness and so on. Indeed Phillipson's (1982) analysis of the political economy of ageing also provides a framework for understanding the political economy of disability, as there are significant parallels.

This can be linked to PCS analysis, as disablism can be seen to operate at all three levels:

P – Personal prejudice against disabled people is relatively commonplace and manifests itself in attitudes of revulsion, dismissiveness, and – paradoxically – also in misplaced charitable concern in which dignity and human rights are exchanged for patronage and good deeds. (This argument will be pursued more fully below.)

C – Cultural values reflect various responses to disability and disabled people, but they are primarily negative in their orientation. Dominant cultural norms are geared towards the able-bodied majority and popular notions present disabled people as either misfits or pathetic victims of personal tragedy. They are also subject to abusive and derogatory treatment in jokes and other forms of humour.

S – Disability is rarely recognized in sociology texts as a dimension of social stratification, and yet it very clearly acts as a social division. This is manifested in the way public services and buildings are provided for the 'general public' but often without due regard for their appropriateness for disabled people, for example, in terms of access or other facilities. Thus, disabled people are structurally/institutionally defined as a marginalized social group – that is, they are not seen as part of the 'general public'.

Voice of experience 6.1

I would have thought that people working in social services would have a good understanding of disability, but that's not always the case. I have been surprised how many people I have worked with who have seemed uncomfortable talking to someone like me in a wheelchair. It's as if they can see the wheelchair but not see me, the person in it. *Len, a hospital social worker*

Oliver (1990) links disablism to the workings of capitalism, the role of wage labour and the pursuit of profit. These are structural factors which underpin the cultural and personal dimensions of disablism and the ideology which sustains them, as we shall see below in the section on the response of the Disabled People's Movement.

PCS analysis is therefore no less applicable to disablism than to the other forms of discrimination and oppression discussed in earlier chapters. One manifestation of disablism is to see disability as a personal tragedy and to focus on the individual level without considering the wider issues of how current social arrangements systematically marginalize and disempower disabled people. Marks comments as follows:

> *Disability* is a highly contested term. Medicine and its allied professions conceptualize disability as damage to a person's body or medical functioning

requiring diagnosis, care or professional treatment. By contrast, the social model of disability argues that 'the problem' should not be located within an individual person, but rather in a 'disabling environment' which excludes and denigrates disabled people.

(Marks, 2000, p. 93)

This passage introduces the notion of a social model of disability which is based on a fundamental distinction between impairment and disability. In the early stages of development of this model, the Union of the Physically Impaired Against Segregation (UPIAS) defined the two terms as follows:

Impairment: lacking part or all of a limb, or having a defective limb, organ or mechanism of the body;

Disability: the disadvantage or restriction of activity caused by a contemporary social organization which takes no or little account of people who have physical impairments and thus excludes them from the mainstream of social activities.

(UPIAS, 1976, pp. 3–4)

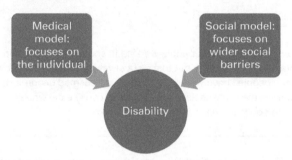

Figure 6.1 Medical vs. social model of disability

More recently, Oliver has explained the social model in the following terms:

The social model of disability does not ignore questions of and concerns relating to impairment and/or the importance of medical and therapeutic treatments. It acknowledges that in many cases, the suffering associated with disabled lifestyles is due primarily to the lack of medical and other services. It is similarly recognized that for many people coming to terms with the consequences of impairment in a society that devalues disabled people and disabled lifestyles is often a personal tragedy. *But the real misfortune is that our society continues to discriminate, exclude and oppress people with impairments.*

(Oliver, 2009, p. 47, emphasis added)

This raises a number of issues for social work staff: are we to be seen as part of the struggle to remove barriers to disability equality or are we ourselves barriers and obstacles due to the tradition of individualism inherent in conventional approaches to disability (Oliver, Sapey and Thomas, 2012) This is a question which will recur in some of the later discussions within this chapter.

To see disability as a matter of personal tragedy or pathology is, to use Ryan's (1988) concept, an example of 'blaming the victim' – that is, the wider social and political dimensions are ignored and the focus remains on a narrow, individualistic level. What is needed, therefore, is a social model of disability or, more specifically, a social oppression model, as this is consistent with the principles of anti-discriminatory practice. Such a model will be explored in more detail in the 'Disabled People's Movement' section below.

Practice focus 6.1

Mary was a social worker who had recently joined a hospital-based team. When she made contact with Mrs Penhaligon to arrange a care package for her return home, she wanted to make sure that her needs were thoroughly assessed. However, Mrs Penhaligon found this intrusive and objected to what she saw as Mary's tendency to patronize her by overemphasizing the difficulties she faced and underestimating her strengths and abilities. This situation began to teach Mary that disability was a much more complex issue than she had originally thought.

A social model of disability underpins the concept of disablism. Parallel with sexism, racism and ageism, as discussed in the preceding chapters, disablism can be seen as a form of discrimination against disabled people premised largely on the stereotypical view that such people are necessarily 'dependent'. A major contributor to this problem is a misguided emphasis on 'helping' people to become more 'independent' by providing care. This view of independence places power in the hands of the professional and can be seen to leave the disabled person more dependent rather than less.

The movement from an individual conception of disability to a social one has many implications for social work and we shall explore these below. However, first, we need to consider how disablism relates to learning disabilities.

For many years issues of mental disorder and mental impairment were dealt with together in policy and legislation under the generic title of 'mental health'. Now, however, they are increasingly being treated as separate entities (although some degree of overlap still remains), with the latter being referred to as 'learning disabilities'.

One significant difference between the two sets of issues is, of course, that the biological basis of mental health problems is disputed, while the physiological basis of learning disability is widely accepted. However, the fact that there is a physiological dimension should not be used as a basis for justifying a medically orientated approach to this area of practice. The critique of the medicalization of disability can also be seen to apply to learning disabilities, as the marginalization and dehumanization inherent in disablism are also applicable to people who have a mental impairment (for example, Down's Syndrome). Many of the points raised in relation to physical disability are therefore also very relevant here, as it can equally be argued that any 'functional disability' engendered by the impairment is amplified and magnified by the social response which attaches negative stereotypes and marginalizes yet another group of citizens from the mainstream of social life. People with a learning disability can therefore be seen to face both disablism generally and, to some degree, discrimination specifically related to issues of learning disability and its confusion with mental 'illness'.

The social response has gone through various stages over the years, forming four distinct models of mental impairment:

The threat to society model   This was a dominant view at the beginning of the twentieth century and was influenced by the eugenics movement who saw mentally impaired people as 'morally defective' and thus a threat to the social order. Thankfully, this view is no longer dominant but is, none the less, still evident in the attitudes of some people.

The medical model   The development of the National Health Service in Britain in the 1940s played a key part in helping the medical profession establish a dominant position and redefine the 'problem' as a medical one, thus requiring the development of a new medical specialism.

The subnormality model   In this model the focus is on educational achievement and the perceived limitations engendered by mental impairment. A key aspect of this model is the measurement of intelligence by means of IQ tests. As IQ is measured in relation to chronological age one implication of this model is that people with a mental impairment are seen as perpetual children. They are subnormal.

The special needs model The focus here is on 'learning difficulties' and attempts are made to achieve the integration of people with a mental impairment into ordinary life as far as possible. However, the emphasis is on special needs and this, in itself, establishes barriers to full integration, especially as the focus remains on the individual and his or her perceived inadequacies rather than on social organization.

Although there is a broad chronological development through from models 1 to 4, this can be misleading, as elements of earlier models persist and influence later models. However, what all these models have in common is a tendency to marginalize and disempower, to a greater or lesser extent, people with a learning disability – that is, they come within the ambit of disablism. Indeed, the discussion below of the 'structure of aiding', is equally applicable in this context. We can question the appropriateness of providing services on an individualistic basis without taking account of the commonalities, of the status of people with learning disabilities as members of a disadvantaged social group whose rights can be affected by negative, demeaning and patronizing social attitudes. What is needed, from an anti-discriminatory point of view, is an approach which does not lose sight of the fact that people with disabilities are indeed *people*, human beings with rights and who should not be arbitrarily discriminated against – just as anti-racist and feminist approaches do in relation to race and gender respectively.

The long-established concept of 'normalization' developed by Wolfensberger (1972) has been very influential in seeking to reintegrate people with learning difficulties into mainstream society. However, the fact that attempts to 'normalize' are directed predominantly at those people excluded, rather than the processes, structures or ideologies which promote such exclusion in the first place, suggests a strong element of 'blaming the victim' and, while that was clearly not Wolfensberger's intention, sadly that is how the idea has often been implemented.

A further criticism of normalization arises in relation to its conception of just what is normal. This is particularly the case in relation to members of ethnic minority communities. For example, Baxter et al. expressed criticism of the tests used in assessment procedures in the learning disability field:

> Such tests are based on the assumption that individuals will identify with images based on white middle-class lifestyles and experiences. Racial stereotyping, inappropriate cultural approaches and language

or communication difficulties further decrease the value of traditional assessments for black and ethnic minority children.

(Baxter et al., 1990, p. 23)

Despite these problems, there does appear to be a growing movement away from a paternalistic 'looking after these poor people' approach towards a genuine aim of empowerment and maximum independence or, to use a concept discussed in Chapter 5 in relation to older people, 'interdependence'.

Once again, this brief analysis most certainly does not do justice to the complexity of the issues, but I hope it has none the less succeeded in its more modest aim of raising awareness of some of the elements involved in developing a truly anti-discriminatory practice in working with people with a learning difficulty.

Of course, with each of the topics discussed in this chapter, we have been able only to skim the surface of each of the areas concerned. And, it should also be recognized, we have by no means explored the full range of possible forms of discrimination. Consider, for example, that it can be shown that people who are dying are often discriminated against (Bevan, 1998), and indeed this is not the only group of people who face discrimination without receiving the same attention or recognition as others.

The aim has been one of flagging up a range of issues which merit further study, debate and development as part of the struggle to achieve a social work practice and theory base premised on principles of challenging discrimination and reducing or removing oppression – in short, principles of emancipatory practice.

The implications for social work

Traditionally, social work with disabled people has a major practical emphasis with a focus on matching available services to assessed need. In this respect there is a strong parallel with traditional social work with older people, as discussed in the previous chapter. Oliver and Sapey (2006) are critical of such an approach, which fails to question what is meant by 'need' and also whether the services on offer are appropriate. They argue that social work with people with disabilities should not be seen as simply a practical matching of resources to needs within a legal and statutory framework. This in itself can be seen as indicative of disablism, in so far as it fails to see disability as a social and political issue and reduces it to a matter of the welfare state providing services for 'dependent' people – thus socially constructing disability as a form of dependency (and hence being part of the problem rather than part of the solution). The 'practical' approach can therefore be understood as an additional form of social oppression that is instrumental in constructing an image of disabled people as helpless and not able to contribute to mainstream society.

This also has implications for those who care for disabled people, as it casts them in a role which can so easily reinforce notions of dependency and pathology. The dominant disablist ideology can have the effect of allowing and encouraging carers to contribute unwittingly to the oppression of the people they are, in most cases, genuinely trying to help.

What all this means is that social workers adopting an anti-discriminatory perspective cannot afford to settle for a 'practical' approach, with an uncritical conception of need. Social work with disabled people must therefore be based on a more sophisticated understanding of the notion of need and the related concept of aiding. What is often overlooked in relation to 'aids to daily living' is the degree of reliance on such aids by 'able-bodied' people. How many could lead 'normal' lives without everyday aids such as pens, cars, telephones, watches, cutlery, reading glasses, stairs and so on? There exists, for each of us, a 'structure of aiding', a set of practical and human support systems which enable us to pursue our day-to-day tasks and lifestyle. For a person with an impairment the structure of such aiding will be different from that of a person who does not have an impairment. However, this is a very different proposition from stating that disabled people need 'aid' (and, by implication, that non-disabled people do not).

The reality of the situation is that all people need some form of assistance or support to participate in mainstream social life. We all have our own requirements, some of which will be common to all, some of which are more individually tailored. However, the way in which such assistance is resourced is a significant issue. For example, government funding is provided in grants and services for individuals and groups, including business interests, and for the general public. That is, aiding is not only for those 'in need'. In fact, the majority of government funding is provided for groups other than people deemed to be 'in need' (spending on roads, defence, mainstream education and so on). It is therefore inappropriate, and indeed stigmatizing, to see the needs of disabled people as 'special', as this draws an arbitrary line between those with an impairment and those without. To see aid as something disabled people need, but which others do not is itself disabling and indeed disablist.

Traditional social work approaches to disability therefore run the risk of falling into this trap.

Oliver went a step further by questioning the traditional helper–helped relationship:

> I would further criticize the 'professionalization' of service for disabled people, on the assumption that the professionals know best what disabled people need and are in charge. The provision of services in such a way is at best patronizing, and at worst further disabling, since disabled people may be pushed into becoming passive recipients of the kinds of services other people think they ought to have.
>
> (Oliver, 1987, p. 18)

What is needed, therefore, is a social work which focuses on partnership rather than paternalism and which sees disabled people not as dependent or childlike, but as an oppressed group who are denied the assistance they need, while assistance for other groups is more freely provided.

Key point 6.1

A key part of anti-discriminatory practice is the need to work in *partnership* – that is, to work *with* the people we are seeking to support, and avoid, where possible, doing things *to* or *for* people. Partnership is a fundamental social work value.

An example of this would be access to public buildings, such as libraries. Steps, where needed, would be provided as a matter of course, whereas adding a ramp for wheelchair access to an existing building is likely to be regarded as a 'special' requirement and may therefore be denied on the grounds of cost. In this way disabled people may be excluded from libraries and other public buildings.

This has a major impact in terms of citizenship and rights. The citizenship of disabled people is undermined by the process illustrated in Figure 6.2, which also shows that it is not the impairment itself which is disabling, but rather the social forces which exclude, marginalize and oppress – disability is the social response to the impairment. The handicap is therefore social rather than physical. This is captured well in Morris's brief but telling comment: 'it is not the inability to walk which disables someone but the steps into the building' (1991, p. 10, cited in Hughes, 1998, p. 77).

This places social workers in a pivotal position within the context of the 'care versus control' dilemma so characteristic of the profession and its undertakings. On the one hand, social work practice can reinforce the traditional individualist model:

> The individual model sees the problems that disabled people experience as being a direct consequence of their impairment. The major task of the professional is therefore to adjust the individual to the particular disabling condition. There are two aspects of this: first there is physical readjustment through rehabilitation programmes designed to return the individual to as near normal a state as possible; and second, there is psychological adjustment which helps the individual to come to terms with physical limitations.
>
> (Oliver and Sapey, 2006, p. 22)

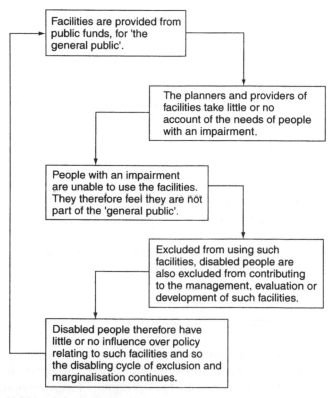

Figure 6.2 Undermining citizenship

The dangers of such a narrow, individualistic approach to social work have already been exemplified in earlier chapters. These include:

- A tendency to 'pathologize', to see the problem as being within the client/service user;
- A tendency to ignore wider cultural and structural factors; and
- Taken-for-granted discriminatory assumptions are not questioned.

In short, it reintroduces many of the weaknesses in theory and practice which radical social work had sought to remove in the 1970s (Bailey and Brake, 1975; Ferguson and Woodward, 2009).

On the other hand, social work practice can confront, challenge and debunk the discriminatory and oppressive basis of the individualist model. Oliver and Sapey (2006) echo Finkelstein's (1981) view that the real problem is:

> one of the need for a change in professional role – the professional must change from expert definer of need and/or rationer of services to become a resource which the disabled person might use as he or she chooses.
>
> (Oliver and Sapey, 2006, p. 180)

A key element in this change is a movement away from a medicalized social work with disabled people towards a practice premised on empowerment and helping disabled people to be as fully in control as possible of their lives and the support they receive. This entails social workers aligning themselves with the Disabled People's Movement and moving away from the traditional ethos of many disability organizations which tend to portray disabled people in largely negative and disempowering ways by using language and imagery which reinforce a sense of tragedy and lack of ability.

A medical model is not only unhelpful through presenting too narrow and negative a picture of disabled people, it also succeeds in relocating power and control in the hands of professionals, particularly medical professionals. This, in turn, plays a significant part in the social construction of dependency (see the discussion of structured dependency in Chapter 5).

What emerges from narrow, individualized and medicalized perspectives is an image of disabled people as individuals for whom a 'cure or care' approach is appropriate. No account is taken of human rights, equality, independence or empowerment. These are all conveniently brushed to one side. It is clear, therefore, that an anti-discriminatory social work practice with disabled people must avoid the dangers of accepting a medical definition of disability or a conception of disabled people as not able to contribute to social life. The focus of practice must not be on the presumed inadequacies of disabled people but on the personal, cultural, structural and physical barriers to taking control of one's own life as far as possible – in short, a social work of empowerment. A significant aspect of this is a shift of focus from charity and compassion to advocacy and rights. As Oliver (1990) has convincingly argued, social policies, including social work itself, should be geared towards alleviating oppression rather than 'compensating' disabled people for their 'tragedy'.

The question of the rights of disabled people is one which has received relatively little attention from social workers or indeed from the state. One factor which can partly explain this disregard for the law and, by extension, the rights of disabled people, is the contradiction between the rights model implicit in this legislation and the medical model which can be seen to underpin the majority of policy and practice in social work agencies. While a medicalized individualist view remains dominant, the emphasis will continue to be on 'adjustment' and treatment rather than empowerment, participation and rights.

This can be taken a step further by arguing that there is a need to change focus so that resources are diverted to dealing with the social causes of disability rather than seeking to deal with the effects. A movement away from a medical model to a social model is a key part of this. As Davis put it:

> For over four centuries in Britain, where disabled people have been among those singled out for legal treatment, we have been dealt with as a problem in need of special treatment and not as equal citizens with a right to full participation in the social mainstream. Countless millions of pounds have been and are spent on research into why we are the way we are, on attempts to cure us, or rehabilitate us, or conductively educate us, or in some other way make us approximate to able-bodiedness, or make us fit into a society designed to serve and perpetuate able-bodied interests. However, when (despite all this effort) we don't quite fit, or can't quite function, or we can't find jobs, millions more pounds are spent on social security, or welfare services, or heart-warming charitable endeavours designed to compensate us in some way for the personal tragedy that has befallen us.
>
> (Davis, 1996, p. 124)

The current emphasis on 'care management' as a key part of the development of community care also retains the influence of the medical model – for example in the assumption that the professional experts know best what the needs of disabled people are. The development of a highly bureaucratic 'managerialism'; as a basis for social policy similarly acts as a potential barrier to moving away from individualized, depoliticized understandings of disability (Finkelstein, 2004; Thompson, 2009a). The move towards personalization is a step in the direction of giving disabled people a voice, of having more say in how they are helped and supported. However, that is no guarantee that the way it is implemented will support an emancipatory, empowering approach to disability.

Anti-disablist practice therefore clearly entails dismantling the traditional medicalized approach and constructing, in its place, a social work practice premised on a social oppression model of disability.

The development of the 'independent living' paradigm (Mercer, 2014) offers social workers a way forward in tackling many of these issues. It focuses on achieving independence and achieving maximization of one's potential. It mainly manifests itself in the establishment of Centres for Independent Living. Basically, such centres examine ways in which policies and services can be changed or created to facilitate maximum independence.

Centres for Independent Living were introduced in the United States in the early 1970s. In the mid-1980s a similar centre was established in Britain, at Ripley in Derbyshire, but with a slightly different focus. The Derbyshire centre is known as a Centre for Integrated Living and constitutes a partnership between local disabled people and the statutory service providers. At its inception the centre aimed to provide a range of services:

1   Maintenance of and updating the Disabled Persons Register.

2   Setting up a county-wide care attendant register.

3   Housing services, from design to direct labour.

4   A coordinated, county-wide accessible transport service.

5   Mixed physical ability, commercially viable workshops.

6   Information, advice and associated support services.

7   Publicity and communications service.

8   Aids and equipment showroom and store.

9 'Halfway House' rehabilitation service.

10 Peer counselling service.

(DCDP, 1985)

This gives an outline of the thinking behind establishing the centre and can act as a model for other areas to follow in seeking an anti-discriminatory approach to social work with disabled people.

Practice focus 6.2

Following the reorganization, a number of working parties were set up to consider the implications of the changes for particular client groups. Tom, the leader of the disability team, was quite insistent that a number of disabled people should be invited to contribute to the working party on disability services. At first he met some resistance from some of his more traditionally minded colleagues. However, he won the argument and the subsequent series of meetings was therefore much more representative and much better informed.

Among the key elements of the CIL and other participatory approaches is a greater control by disabled people themselves over their lives and circumstances. But it must be recognized that poverty acts as a major limitation on such control. Without the financial wherewithal to build an independent lifestyle, people with an impairment will remain, to a certain extent at least, disabled victims of a sociopolitical handicap, rather than a physical one.

It is also important to recognize the twofold relationship between poverty and disability. On the one hand, disability consigns people with an impairment to a position of low income and, on the other hand, poverty can, in itself, be seen as a major cause of disability (Oliver, 2009). The links between disability and the economy will be discussed in the following section but the point to note at this stage is the significance of poverty as a restrictive factor in the lives of disabled people. This places issues of welfare rights advocacy on the social work agenda as well as steps towards improved employment opportunities.

Again the question of rights arises and this is indeed a major issue for anti-disablist social work – the development of an approach in which strategies of intervention address rights, independent living and participation, rather than simply adjustment or rehabilitation. This involves challenging discriminatory and oppressive structures, practices and attitudes both within and outside social work organizations.

Voice of experience 6.2

My approach to working with disabled people has evolved significantly over time. I began by doing straightforward assessments to help people get services. But over time I got interested in rights and advocacy issues and ended up specializing in that area because I was so dissatisfied with just being a rationer of scarce resources, while so many key issues for disabled people were not being addressed. *Fiona, the manager of a disability rights service*

The British Council of Organisations of Disabled People (BCODP – now the UK Disabled People's Council: UKDPC) played a key role in campaigning for anti-discrimination legislation. Although the Disability Discrimination Act 1995 and the Equality Act 2010 have gone some way towards tackling discrimination, they leave many aspects of disablism untouched. As Chadwick (1996) argued in response to the implementation of the Disability Discrimination Act, the legislation perpetuates an individualist model of disablement and fails to address the social basis of disability and the consequences of a society geared towards the able-bodied majority.

The anti-disablist response: the Disabled People's Movement

'The Disabled People's Movement' is a generic term used to describe the politicization of disability issues and the construction and consolidation of an approach which avoids, and indeed undermines, the traditional model of disability. The movement promotes, as we have seen, a model of disability as a form of social oppression rather than personal misfortune or 'tragedy'. It attempts to move away from forms of practice which:

● fail to acknowledge the significant physical and social barriers faced by disabled people;

● regard disabled people as 'sick' or necessarily in need of care and attention;

● reinforce unduly negative images and perceptions of disabled people;

● have a tendency to infantilize and patronize; and

● assume dependency rather than promote empowerment.

These points represent some of the various dimensions of oppression experienced by disabled people which are rarely, if ever, acknowledged by traditional approaches to disability.

The individualist approach which constructs disability as a matter of personal tragedy is a model the Disabled People's Movement seeks to replace with a more politically informed strategy that does not neglect the significance of wider social and economic factors (Barnes and Mercer, 2010). The types of changes needed are highlighted in the following passage from Hughes:

> If we were to adopt the view that disability is a form of social oppression, how might this be translated into policies? It would perhaps lead to social policies which focused on disabled people as both the collective 'victim' and survivors of a prejudiced and discriminatory society rather than as individual victims of circumstance. Such social (rather than medical) policies would thus be geared to the alleviation of oppression rather than the compensation of individuals, and would lead to structural interventions such as the redistribution of resources, changing the physical environment, and equal rights policies.
>
> (Hughes, 1998, p. 77)

Finkelstein (1981) linked disability with social and political factors by tracing the historical development of the role of people with an impairment in the economy. Prior to the Industrial Revolution, such people were able to contribute to production in cottage and family-based industries, as machines were relatively simple and easily adapted. Modern industrial methods, however, are less easily adapted, are located away from the home and involve a division of labour, thus excluding significant numbers of people with impairments from the labour market and consequently from the opportunity to be financially self-sufficient. Dependency is therefore caused not by the impairment itself but by the social arrangements which take no account of the needs of people with an impairment.

Oliver (1990) adopted a similar line of argument in linking the exclusion of disabled people to the workings of capital. He put forward the idea that there are both economic and ideological reasons for capitalist social relations to marginalize disabled people. Economically, they contribute to the 'reserve army of labour' in much the same way as women, ethnic minorities and older people. That is, disabled people provide the capitalist economy with a degree of flexibility in managing fluctuations in the demand for labour. Ideologically, the inferior position of disabled people serves 'as a warning to those unable or unwilling to work' (Oliver, 1990, p. 70).

There are therefore structural reasons for the inequitable position of disabled people in western societies; it is no coincidence or historical accident – it is, in part at least, the outcome of historic material forces not unconnected with the nature of the capitalist economic system (**S**) and the ideology of competitiveness and individualism (**C**) which helps to sustain it. This ideology is instrumental in constructing disabled people in negative terms, as people with problems – or even as people who *are* problems. Thus, this dominant ideology of disability focuses specifically on the negative aspects of impairment and thereby presents a biased and unbalanced picture of disabled people. Indeed, it is a recurring theme in the literature on disablism that dominant ideologies of disability have a tendency to:

- stereotype disabled people as passive, dependent and in need of care (and sympathy);

- emphasize the negative effects of impairment; and

- treat disabled people as problems (rather than as people with problems caused by the social arrangements which undermine their autonomy and exclude them from mainstream society).

It is precisely this negative, demeaning and thus discriminatory, perspective on disability that the Disabled People's Movement is determined to fight and ultimately eliminate. The dehumanization inherent in disablism is an important target for the attentions of those committed to achieving equality and human rights.

Such dehumanization manifests itself in the language used to describe, or refer to disabled people, as Brisenden has helpfully indicated in the following passage:

> To begin with, we are not 'the disabled'. We are disabled people or even people with disabilities. It is important that we do not allow ourselves to be dismissed as if we all come under this one great metaphysical category 'the disabled'. The effect of this is a depersonalization, a sweeping dismissal of our individuality, and a right to be seen as people with our own uniqueness rather than the anonymous constituents of a category or group. These words that lump us all together – 'the disabled', 'spina bifida', 'tetra-plegic', 'muscular dystrophy' – are nothing more than terminological rubbish bins into which all the important things such as people get thrown away.
>
> (Brisenden, 1986, p. 174)

This powerfully worded statement captures well the impact an ill-considered use of language can have on disabled people. A key factor in the struggle against disablism is therefore the development of a greater sensitivity to the discriminatory effects of language and the construction of a more appropriate vocabulary of empowerment.

Much work remains to be done before equality can become a reality for disabled people. The 'charitable' approach which presents disabled people as objects of pity and sympathy has a long legacy, and so its influence and consequences will not wither away overnight. This is especially the case when we consider that this approach has not developed in isolation but is, rather, a reflection of the broader economic and political sphere which values people's contribution to society in terms of the part they play in the production process and the creation of wealth.

It is partly in recognition of these wider aspects that the Disabled People's Movement has sought to politicize disability issues by, for example, seeing them as a civil rights matter, a struggle for the replacement of charity with rights, rather than simply a call for more or better services. We are witnessing a 'paradigm shift', a major change in how we think of disability and how we respond to it. What is called for is not a modification of the existing approach or 'paradigm' but rather a completely new paradigm which focuses not on individual tragedy or 'special' needs, but more appropriately on the barriers to empowerment and self-realization that a disabling society places before those citizens who have an impairment.

The Disabled People's Movement seeks to reconstruct the image of disabled people in the eyes of mainstream society. They seek to establish the recognition that all people require some form of aiding to live satisfactory day-to-day lives and we should not discriminate against people with an impairment simply because the aiding they require is different from the majority (that is, different not special). It is an arrogant and inaccurate assumption to see disabled people as those in need of aid as opposed to able-bodied people who are not.

This more radical approach casts down a considerable challenge to social workers, as the actions of social work staff cannot be neutral – they will either follow traditional lines and thus reinforce the oppression of disabled people or they will challenge traditional methods by contributing to the emancipation and empowerment of people with disabilities.

Multiple oppressions

So far in this chapter the emphasis has been specifically on the oppression inherent in the social response to disability. The aim of this section, then, is to widen the focus somewhat in order to consider how disablism intersects with other forms of discrimination and oppression. This is, of course, a complex and multifaceted area and so, once again, it must be recognized that the discussion here is exploratory and far from comprehensive.

Disablism has a particular link with ageism, as the incidence of impairment is greater in the older age groups than in the population as a whole. This statistical point is often misconstrued, and it emerges as an aspect of ageist ideology: the false assumption that old age itself is a form of disability or impairment (see Chapter 5). However, what does in fact occur is that very many older people suffer the dual oppression of a combination of ageism and disablism; they are marginalized and negatively stereotyped on both counts. This can have the effect of amplifying the discriminatory impact of both forms of oppression. An example of this would be attitudes towards sexuality. As has been noted in Chapter 5, ageism constructs older people as asexual and thus presents sexual activity in old age as 'deviant'. A similar process occurs in relation to disabled people who are also assumed to be asexual. A disabled older person therefore faces an even greater attitudinal barrier to fulfilling sexual desire.

Many other examples could be given but I hope the point is clear that age and disability are not simply separate social forces – they converge and overlap in many significant ways which will have important implications for older disabled people. One result of this is that social workers who work with older people should be conscious not only of issues of ageism but also of disablism.

Gender also features as a significant dimension of the experience of disabled people. The work of Lonsdale (1990) helped to put the complex intertwining of gender and disability on the agenda. She explored a number of important themes, one of which was that of dependency:

> Dependency has particular implications for women because of the important part which gender plays in determining whether someone is expected or encouraged, or indeed is even allowed to be independent. Since women are encouraged to play a more dependent role in society than men, women with disabilities often have a particular struggle to achieve control over their own destinies, although they are sometimes 'allowed' out of the passive and dependent female role.
>
> (Lonsdale, 1990, pp. 10–11)

Social expectations of dependency apply to women in general within the strictures of patriarchy, but for disabled women the additional stereotyped equation of disability with dependency further promotes an image of disabled women as people who need to be 'looked after'. It does not, then, take much imagination to see the impact of this as negative and limiting. Similarly, Lonsdale argues that women are 'invisible' in the majority of accounts of disability and so issues of gender and sexism are not paid adequate attention, even though far more women than men have disabilities (but see Robertson, 2014, for a discussion about how the specific experiences of disabled men are also neglected).

Practice focus 6.3

Paula was a student on placement at a disability resource centre where a range of advice, information and advocacy services was provided. Her main task was to interview people who sought a service, and help to determine the most appropriate response to their request. In supervision Paula and her practice teacher discussed her work in some detail. From this it emerged that Paula was doing very well indeed in general terms. However, what also emerged was that she appeared to be operating within stereotypical expectations as far as gender was concerned. For example, in her dealings with men, Paula often addressed employment issues, but rarely did so with the women who sought her help. In her anxiety to avoid relying on disablist assumptions she had neglected to take account of gender.

One account which has recognized the intersection of sexism and disablism is that of Sheldon:

> There is little recognition from those who experience disability oppression and those who experience sexist oppression that their concerns are similar (Sheldon, 1999). Disabled women are said to fall between two stools – peripheral as women in the disabled people's movement, invisible as disabled people in the women's movement (Lloyd, 2001). Thus, the gendered nature of disability is not given a high priority, giving rise to some specific concerns for disabled women.
>
> (Sheldon, 2014, p. 70)

Gender roles therefore take on an extra significance from the standpoint of disability and place extra pressures and restrictions on disabled women in particular. In short, sexism amplifies the negative effects of disablism and disablism exacerbates the negative impact of sexism. While the focus of scholarship in this area has understandably been on disabled women, we should also note that sexism can be oppressive for disabled men by placing them under pressure to fulfil conventional expectations of masculinity.

A social work of empowerment is also a relevant issue in considering how disability and race combine to provide another example of interlocking and mutually reinforcing oppressions. Over the years there has been a notable, and very welcome, growth in literature addressing issues of anti-racist social work, but sadly anti-racism in the context of social work with disabled people has yet to receive adequate attention. The dynamics of racism and disablism as a combination of oppressions remains a neglected area and one which clearly merits further research and the articulation of a coherent theory base. Banton and Singh (2014) recognize the need for further work in this area and offer some useful pointers towards a more adequate theoretical understanding of the issues. They argue that disablism should not be seen in isolation from other forms of discrimination. This reinforces the point I made earlier that exploring how different forms of discrimination interact should not be a matter of adding them together in a simplistic way – they are dimensions of experience that interact in complex and subtle ways. None the less, despite the relative lack of material to inform our understanding of such multiple oppressions, the significance of such combinations can be readily appreciated and their implications for practice can at least begin to be addressed.

Towards anti-disablist practice

This chapter has outlined the development of a new approach to social work with disabled people which is quite radically different from traditional perspectives. Much of the change has stemmed from disabled people who have sought to rework the helper–helped relationship. The movement remains a 'consumer-led' one, but this is not to say that social workers do not have a major contribution to make. The remainder of this chapter is therefore a set of suggestions for taking steps towards an anti-discriminatory social work with disabled people. These are by no means the only steps, but will, I hope, none the less help social workers to engage with the issues and determine, in more detail, the route they wish to follow.

1 Disabled people are people first. This may seem straightforward but it is something which is not always recognized in interactions between social workers and disabled clients. The history of social work intervention with disabled people has not been a particularly happy one. Much of the criticism has stemmed from the view that the focus tends to be on the disability rather than on the person (as per the medical

model – see point 2 below). Anti-discriminatory practice must be based on seeing the person first, before the disability.

2   Social work with disabled people has for many years been dominated by the medical model. The social work task has been seen as a para-medical or ancillary task geared towards caregiving and rehabilitation. The more critical approach to disability developed by Oliver, Finkel-stein, Sapey and so on is now capable of creating a more adequate theory base, so that the medical model is not needed to make sense of people's experiences of disability. Treating disabled people as if they were ill or necessarily in need of medical supervision is dehumanizing and oppressive. Anti-discriminatory practice must therefore aim for a 'demedicalization' of social work.

3   Traditional social work with disabled people is premised on an indi-vidual model of personal tragedy and efforts are geared towards the individual for his or her lack of functional ability. However, this has now been challenged by a social oppression model of disability which emphasizes the personal, cultural, structural and environmental barri-ers that prevent disabled people from participating fully in mainstream social, political and economic life. In fact, the individual model is seen as a further barrier to self-realization, as it translates issues of human rights into matters of care and rehabilitation. Anti-discriminatory prac-tice must therefore be based on a social, rather than an individual, model of disability.

4   Following on from this, it needs to be recognized that the service disa-bled people's organizations are looking for is one based on rights rather than (or as well as) compassion, on a commitment to assisting disabled people to achieve maximum independence, rather than to 'looking after them'. If we fail to recognize this, our efforts to help – however genuine and humane in intention – can be disabling and thus discriminatory and oppressive in their outcomes. Social work has an important role in helping disabled people to assert their own choices and thus move to a less dependent role. This can be a key part in the development of anti-disablist practice.

5   The dominance of disablist ideology which constructs disabled people as passive and pitiful victims of personal tragedy is reflected in, and reinforced by, the language commonly used to refer to disabled peo-ple. It is therefore important to ensure that discriminatory and dehu-manizing language is avoided and discouraged. Depersonalizing terms such as 'the disabled', 'the handicapped' or 'spastic' not only

contribute to the oppression of disabled people but also legitimate such oppression by making it seem natural, 'normal' and a straightforward part of everyday life. A more sensitive and positive use of language is therefore called for.

6 Part of the discriminatory ideology of disablism is the tendency to see disabled people as those in need of aid as opposed to 'normal' people who do not need such aid. This is an oppressive and divisive myth which isolates disabled people from the mainstream of society. By disguising the assistance all people rely on and the public resources which finance much of such assistance, the type of aiding required by people with an impairment appears to be 'special' and costly – and is therefore vulnerable to cutbacks and rationing and seen as a privilege rather than a right. It therefore needs to be remembered that aiding is for all and therefore the needs of people with an impairment are different rather than a 'special case'. Social workers can play a part in drawing attention to this and thus contribute to 'destigmatizing' disability.

7 Given that aiding is for all, we are all 'dependent' to some extent on assistance. The fact that such a reliance is exaggerated and overemphasized in the stereotype of disability is a further dimension of disablist ideology. It is therefore important that social work intervention has the effect of promoting independence as far as possible. There is a danger that an uncritical social work practice informed by received ideas will assume dependency to be the norm and thus run the risk of creating such dependency by establishing a 'self-fulfilling prophecy'. What is needed therefore is a practice based on partnership rather than paternalism.

Key point 6.2

Stereotypes of disability and disabled people are very common and very influential. We therefore have to get past such stereotypes and develop a fuller, more sophisticated understanding of disability and the powerful role of disablism in society.

---

8 A focus on independence is precisely the strategy of Centres for Independent Living (CILs). These centres involve putting power and control into the hands of disabled people themselves. This is, of course, entirely consistent with anti-disablism and a movement to

be supported and encouraged. The development of anti-discriminatory practice will therefore be hindered by a traditional approach which sees the social work task in predominantly casework terms and shies away from community involvement or wider-scale initiatives. CILs should not be seen as developments ripe for professional colonization, but nor should they be seen as a separate venture largely unconnected with the aims, values and interests of social workers.

9 The casework approach has also tended to produce an emphasis on practical tasks, a very pragmatic sorting out services and benefits approach. It is no doubt partly due to this that social work with disabled people has tended to be seen as a lower status branch of social work, often consigned to unqualified staff. Social work with disabled people is a professional endeavour which requires commitment and a range of skills, including assessment, negotiation, advocacy, counselling and so on. Helping to overcome oppression is a skilled and demanding task and should not be viewed as a subordinate, lower status aspect of social work – as that would itself be a disablist assumption to make.

10 Perhaps the central concept in the development of anti-disablist practice is that of empowerment. Traditional approaches to disability continue to disempower people with an impairment, to deprive them of aspects of control over their own lives. They are disenfranchised by marginalization, isolation and dehumanization – at a personal level through prejudice and misdirected pity; at a cultural level through negative stereotypes and values; at a structural level through a society dominated by capitalist notions of 'survival of the fittest' and charity for those who are 'handicapped' from competing. Empowerment amounts to working alongside disabled people to help overcome and challenge the oppression they experience. This involves counselling geared towards confidence-boosting and similar measures on the one hand, and advocacy and the promotion of citizenship on the other.

Social work has never been a static entity and is therefore no stranger to change and innovation. However, it must be recognized that the changes required to develop anti-disablist social work practice are, in many ways, major and radical. This does not mean it cannot be done; indeed it is already under way in some areas. But this is clearly a major challenge for social work and one to which I very much hope we are able to rise.

Food for thought

- Do you have a disability or do you know someone who has a disability? If so, can you see how social attitudes and expectations affect the experience of disability?
- What stereotypes of disabled people can you identify? How can you ensure that you do not allow these to affect your practice?
- How can social workers be involved in contributing to the empowerment of disabled people rather than making them dependent?

Further resources

Oliver, Sapey and Thomas (*Social Work with Disabled People*, 2012) is an updated version of a classic text which has had a profound influence on social work thinking. Other important works involving leading thinker and activist, Mike Oliver, include: Oliver and Barnes (*The New Politics of Disablement*, 2012); and Oliver (*Understanding Disability: From Theory to Practice*, 2009). Barnes and Mercer (*Exploring Disability*, 2010) and Swain et al. (*Disabling Barriers – Enabling Environments*, 2014) are also both important texts.

Sapey ('Disability', 2002) and Sapey ('Impairment, Disability and Loss: Reassessing the Rejection of Loss', 2004) are two important contributions to our understanding of the relationship between disability and loss. Clements and Read (*Disabled People and European Human Rights*, 2003) provide a helpful guide to the implications of the Human Rights Act 1998 for disabled people. Hans and Patri (2003) discusses women, disability and identity.

Other important texts include: Cameron (*Disability Studies: A Student's Guide*, 2014); Goodley (*Disability Studies: An Interdisciplinary Introduction*, 2011); and Shakespeare (*Disability Rights and Wrongs Revisited*, 2013). Also, the journal, *Disability and Society*, is a regular source of relevant articles.

CHAPTER 7

SEXUALITY AND HETEROSEXISM

CHAPTER OVERVIEW

In this chapter you will:

- Learn about how a person's sexual orientation or identity can form the basis of discrimination in a variety of ways
- Appreciate how much harm such discrimination can do
- Explore the implications of such matters for professional practice

Introduction

Since the 1980s we have seen an increased awareness of issues of sexual identity and the discriminatory and negative treatment of gay, lesbian, bisexual and transgender people. Such discrimination has increasingly been recognized as unjust and, since the implementation of the Employment Equality (Sexual Orientation) Regulations 2003 and the Equalities Act (Sexual Orientation) Regulations 2007, has featured in a high proportion of equality or diversity policies. The implementation of the Equality Act 2010 has also offered a further degree of protection from discrimination on the grounds of their sexual orientation. As we have noted, there is much more to anti-discriminatory practice than legal provision and compliance, but the legal changes are none the less to be welcomed.

In this chapter we will explore the nature of discrimination on the grounds of sexual orientation (known as heterosexism), its implications for social work, efforts to challenge such discrimination and guidelines for trying to ensure that our anti-discriminatory practice does not neglect matters of sexuality and sexual orientation.

It is important to note that sexuality is often a feature of social policy even if it is not directly or openly mentioned. As Carabine comments:

> Significantly, social policy does not have to be specifically concerned with sexuality for it to 'speak' of sexuality and for it to regulate sexual relations and behaviour. Social policies about, for example, housing, health,

education, social exclusion, income support or parenting can also contain assumptions and convey messages about acceptable and normal sexual relations and practices as taking place within a two-parent married family … [W]hat we 'do' sexually, our sexual relationships and how we experience our sexuality can be affected by policy and welfare interventions which at first glance have nothing to do with sexuality. In policy, welfare analyses and practice, sexuality is usually taken as given, as something that 'just is', and welfare subjects are assumed to be universally heterosexual. The idea of heterosexuality is left unproblematized and unquestioned.

(Carabine, 2004a, pp. 2–3)

Ironically, while sexuality often features implicitly in these ways, there is often no explicit focus on sexuality issues, leaving many social work situations open to distortion because of a reliance on oversimplified, 'commonsense' understandings of how sexuality features in people's lives. This is a dangerous position to be in because of such distortion in general, but there are also specific issues of discrimination to consider – that is, issues that arise in relation to the tendency to see heterosexuality as the valued norm and other forms of sexuality as problematic or even 'unhealthy'. This chapter therefore explores how we need a more sophisticated understanding of sexuality to make sure that we are not unwittingly reinforcing heterosexist norms and assumptions.

What is heterosexism?

The heightened awareness of discrimination on the grounds of sexuality has been recognized in the coining of a new term in the anti-discriminatory vocabulary – 'heterosexism', which can be explained in the following terms:

Heterosexism reflects the dominance of the world-view in which heterosexuality is used as the standard against which all people are measured; everyone is assumed to be heterosexual unless proven otherwise, and anyone not fitting into this pattern is considered to be abnormal, sick, morally corrupt and inferior. The assumption of heterosexuality and its superiority is perpetuated through its institutionalization within laws, media, religions and language, which either actively discriminate against non-heterosexuals or else render them invisible through silence. Just as the concepts of racism and sexism have helped us to understand the oppression of black people and women, so the concept of heterosexism has assisted us in theorizing lesbian and gay oppression.

(Wise, 2000, p. 154)

As Wise implies, there are strong parallels between heterosexism and other forms of discrimination (not least the applicability of PCS analysis). For example, there is a reliance on biological (or pseudo-biological) explanations of why same-sex relationships are not 'natural' and are therefore seen as 'deviant' and to be discouraged. However, to argue that one form of sexuality is natural while another is not is a matter of ideological construction rather than biological explanation. It amounts, as Hocquenghem has pointed out, to arguing that: 'Some of us are part of nature, and some not' (1978, p. 48). The oppressive implications of this assumption are, of course, vast, and so it is not too difficult to appreciate the negative impact of this aspect of heterosexism. Sanders highlights the costs of heterosexism (although she uses the term, 'homophobia') for young people in particular:

What are the costs of homophobia?

• Alcohol and drug misuse – blocking out the pain

• Truancy as students seek to escape from persecution

• Giving up on academic achievements as students find they are unable to work effectively in their environment

• Promiscuous sexual practices leading to early pregnancies due to confusion and internalized homophobia.

(Sanders, 2008, p. 7)

A further parallel is the alienation, marginalization and destructive humour to which gay, lesbian, bisexual and transsexual people are subjected. A very negative and discriminatory attitude is even witnessed within the so-called caring professions. For example, Munro and McCulloch, in a text written for social workers, commented that: 'Most lesbians are content to keep their homosexual inclinations hidden from general view and it is only the most psychopathic among them who make a show of their abnormality' (1969, p. 157). This comment was made many years ago, but we should not be complacent in assuming that the problems no longer apply.

One of the factors which can be seen to underlie heterosexism is a degree of paranoia, a fear that an acceptance of homosexuality will undermine family values to the extent that the social and moral order will be seriously weakened. Another term that is commonly used is that of 'homophobia'. Literally, phobia means fear, and so it is used to mean fear of homosexuality and then extended to mean hatred of homosexuality (as we shall see in Chapter 8, there is a parallel here with Islamophobia).

Homophobia is therefore a key aspect of heterosexism. It reflects the common tendency for many people to fear (and then to hate) things that they do not understand, phenomena that are outside their usual sphere of reference. These comments reflect Hocquenghem's view that: 'The problem is not so much homosexual desire as the fear of homosexuality' (1978, p. 35). Such fear and paranoia can lead to people having to conceal their sexual identity and make a secret of their personal, intimate relationships or even deny them for fear of reprisal, ridicule or some other form of social sanction. The negative well-being can therefore be quite considerable.

'Homosexuality' literally means sexuality involving same-sex relations. However, this very straightforward, literal definition gives us no sense of the intense disapproval, antipathy and even hostility towards people who in some way depart from the assumed natural order of heterosexuality (opposite-sex relations). In considering the significance of discrimination in people's lives, there is therefore much we can learn from exploring how oppression features in the lives of gay, lesbian, bisexual and transgender people.

Voice of experience 7.1

I worked with a teenage boy once who was having all sorts of problems in his life. He had been received into care as a result of physical abuse. When I met him it quickly became apparent to me that he was gay. Nowhere in his extensive file did it say that, and his foster carers said they were not aware of this either. I really felt for him. After all the various people who had been trying to help him, it seems I was the only one who acknowledged his sexuality. No wonder he started talking much more openly to me than he had to anyone else.

Sanders makes the important point that we should not see people who do not fit in with the heterosexual norm as members of a homogeneous group. She emphasizes the need to recognize the diversity of the people involved:

Lesbians, gay men, bisexuals and trans people are Black, White, dual-heritage, daughters, sons, aunts, mothers, sisters, brothers, fathers, uncles, nephews, nieces, friends, colleagues, workers, non-waged, students, teachers, customers, non-disabled, Jewish, Hindu, Sikh, Muslim, Christian, of all religions and none, old and young, women and men, live in both rural and urban areas and represent every political perspective.

(Sanders, 2008, p. 3)

Heterosexism will therefore apply alongside other forms of discrimination. We shall return to this point below under the heading 'Multiple oppressions'.

The implications for social work

For many years issues of sexuality were seen as mental health matters (it was only in 1973 that homosexuality ceased to be categorized as a mental illness). Partly this was because same-sex relationships were seen as unnatural, deviations from the norm of 'healthy' heterosexuality. The first implication for social work, then, is the need not to pathologize same-sex relations and to recognize the discrimination involved in the assumption that such relations represent a problem to be solved rather than a reflection of the diversity and fluidity of sexuality.

Discrimination against gay, lesbian, bisexual and transsexual people can be seen to have two major sets of implications, one in relation to staff/ service providers and the other in relation to clients/service users. I shall consider each in turn.

Staff experiences

One common assumption which can have a profoundly discriminatory effect on staff is the false notion that homosexuals are a threat to children. It is commonly assumed by many people that homosexuals regard children as valid objects of sexual desire. This is reflected in, for example, the French use of the term 'pédéraste', which literally means 'lover of children', to refer to homosexuals in general – and this is even confirmed in the dictionary definition (*Le Petit Robert*). It is therefore important that such discriminatory assumptions at the cultural level are not allowed to influence our thoughts and actions at the personal level. The risk any individual poses to children is something that needs to be assessed very carefully in each case and is not something that should be distorted by inaccurate and discriminatory generalizations or stereotypes.

However, this is not the only way in which staff employed in social work can face heterosexist discrimination. As a consultant and training facilitator I have come across a worryingly wide range of examples of discrimination against staff – whether from clients or carers, managers, colleagues within their own agency or colleagues from other agencies. I have also come across many examples of heterosexual staff who have faced negative responses because they have been supportive of gay rights.

Client experiences

The irrational view of homosexuality as a threat is indicative of the paranoia which both reflects and reinforces heterosexist ideology. This ideology is also apparent in some social work dealings with clients. In 1989 Webb argued that: 'All the while social workers, home helps and so on at best assume clients are heterosexual and at worst make homophobic comments' (p. 21). I would like to think that the situation has improved since then, but it would be naïve to assume that such attitudes are no longer part of social work and social care. An insensitive, ill-informed social work practice can therefore not only fail to play a part in tackling the oppression of heterosexism, but can also actually contribute significantly to such oppression.

Practice focus 7.1

Len was an experienced social worker in an emergency duty team. One night he was called out to deal with a situation in which Mrs Todd, an elderly woman, was in need of urgent support. As a result of this referral, Len contacted Mrs Todd's son, Alan. Alan expressed a willingness to care for his mother, but explained that this might cause friction as he had had little contact with her since he 'came out' and she told him he was no longer her son. The realization that Alan was gay had a profound effect on Len – it generated very strong negative feelings in him. Some days later Len reflected on the situation and his feelings, and felt very guilty about his negative reaction. He began to realize just how deeply ingrained discriminatory feelings and prejudices can be.

The development of anti-discriminatory practice must therefore be based on a greater understanding of homosexuality and heterosexism. This is particularly the case in relation to children's services, in England and Wales, at least, where the Children Act 1989 expects the self-esteem needs of gay young people to be addressed. Shortly after the implementation of the Act, Sone explained this as follows:

[Social services] departments must come out of the closet and place the needs of lesbian and gay young people firmly on the agenda. The potential for this revolution can be found in The Children Act. The guidance on family placements states that when leaving care 'the needs and concerns of gay young men must be recognized and approached sympathetically'.

(Sone, 1991, p. 12)

It is to be hoped, of course, that anti-discriminatory practice will amount to more than a sympathetic approach, as this has patronizing and tokenistic connotations. However, as part of a broader-based commitment to fighting oppression, this is a worthwhile start.

Sanders also comments on the impact of heterosexism on children and young people (although much of what she describes can also apply to adults):

> Here's what's happening to our young people in schools. This is what they're facing:
>
> - Sixty-five per cent of lesbian and gay pupils have experienced homophobic bullying
>
> - Of those, 92 per cent (143,000) have experienced verbal homophobic bullying, 41 per cent (64,000) physical bullying and 17 per cent (26,000) death threats
>
> - 97 per cent of pupils hear derogatory phrases such as 'dyke', 'queer' and 'rug-muncher' used in school
>
> - Half of teachers fail to respond to homophobic language when they hear it
>
> - Thirty per cent of lesbian and gay pupils say that adults – teachers or support staff – are responsible for homophobic incidents in their school
>
> - Less than a quarter of schools have told pupils that homophobic bullying is wrong (Hunt and Jensen, 2007).
>
> (Sanders, 2008, p. 6)

(See also Ellison and Gunstone, 2009, for statistics about the negative impact of heterosexism.) These figures paint a worrying picture and one which reflects the importance of the **C** level of cultural assumptions and frameworks of meaning – discrimination arising not simply from personal prejudice, but from cultural formations into which we are socialized from childhood onwards, and which are, in themselves linked to structural relations that allocate people to dominant and subordinate (or 'subaltern') groups.

Key point 7.1

Attitudes to non-mainstream forms of sexuality have changed over the years and there is now far less overt discrimination towards, and rejection of, people who are gay, lesbian, bisexual or transgender. However, we should not allow that progress to lure us into complacency. Discrimination on the grounds of sexuality remains commonplace and can be highly destructive.

Canavan and Prior (2008) give us further insights into the significance of cultural factors, as manifested in peer pressure. They argue that many young people are likely to feel coerced into sexual activity due to pressure from other young people. If their preferences around sexuality place them in a minority, they may experience difficulties that require additional support from understanding adults. They go on to say that other young people may start to question their own sexual orientation, and this too can lead to potential problems:

> young people who have difficulty in acknowledging a sexual orientation other than straight, may have behavioural problems which may result in them coming into care. If the young person has experienced same-sex feelings or relationships they will need sensitive work and support. They may experience victimization by other children, compounding an already fragile sexual identity. If staff have not looked at the issue in training they may believe that there is something wrong with being lesbian or gay and pathologize the young person rather than offer them the support which they need.
>
> (Canavan and Prior, 2008, p. 334)

While it is clearly the case that heterosexism raises significant issues for social work with children and young people, we should also note that our concerns about such discrimination should not be limited to children's services. Consider, for example, the following scenarios, each of which raises challenges for social workers committed to anti-discriminatory practice:

- Tom had been diagnosed as having a bipolar disorder some years ago. His condition was largely controlled by medication, but a significant thorn in his side was that there were people in his workplace who taunted him about being gay. They were quite vicious at times and this made it difficult to keep his emotions under control.

- Mrs Hobson 'came out' as bisexual after her husband died. This created a great deal of bad feeling at the day centre she attended and she felt she was no longer welcome there. She had hoped that people would be supportive of her through her grief, and so she was devastated by this response.

- When Colin, their son with learning disabilities, seemed to be forming a romantic attachment to another man with learning disabilities who attended the same work skills development scheme, Mr and Mrs Pearson threatened to make a formal complaint on the grounds that their son was likely to be sexually abused.

● Marina had lived with her lesbian lover for several years and was hit very hard when she died. She felt very unsupported when most people reacted as if she had had a relatively minor loss (a flatmate), rather than a major loss of her lover and life partner. She had had previous minor bouts of depression, but she found this whole experience quite traumatic and became severely depressed to the extent that she needed hospitalization.

The anti-heterosexist response

The term 'Gay liberation movement' has now become part of our every-day vocabulary rather than a specialist political term. This has been a successful movement in some ways, in so far as overt discrimination is far less prevalent than was previously the case and there are now legal pro-tections in place. However, we should not allow this relative success to obscure the fact that we still have a long way to go when it comes to sexu-alities equality.

A key part of the gay liberation movement has been political protests and campaigning (the work of Stonewall, for example: www.stonewall .org.uk). Changes in cultural politics – for example, how people are pre-sented in the media – have also played a part (Gauntlett, 2002). However, developments in theoretical understanding have also played a central role in helping us to move away from heterosexist assumptions. This approach to theorizing has come to be known as 'queer theory'. Hodges describes it in the following terms:

> Queer Theory is fundamentally about power, politics and activism. In particular, it focuses on the ways in which our most private understandings of who we are, who we desire, and who we love, of acceptance and rejection, sameness and difference, are shaped, moulded and regulated by relations of language, power and authority. In short, Queer Theory focuses upon how power gets inside our bodies, our 'hearts' and our heads. It is above all oppositional – opposing all forms of oppression including the ways that seemingly liberatory categories, especially 'lesbian', 'gay', 'bisexual' and 'trans', may themselves become tied to (oppressive) regulatory regimes and practices.
>
> (Hodges, 2008, p. 8)

The term 'queer', as used in this context, is an example of 'reclaiming the language' – that is, of terms that are used in a discriminatory way being redefined in more positive terms as part of a political statement reaffirming equality (Thompson, 2012). Lance explains this as follows:

> to be queer in the old usage was first to be excluded from what is 'proper', and then to be reviled for it. To call oneself queer in the new usage is to endorse that exclusion and to turn the evaluation on its head, to embrace difference as a challenge to what is regarded as proper.
>
> (Lance, 2005, p. 182)

Queer theory derives from the work of Butler (2006) whose work, in turn, owes much to the writings of the French philosopher and social theorist, Michel Foucault (especially Foucault, 1979). Butler argues that gender is not something that we *are* (as a result of being a man or a woman). Rather, gender is what we 'do' – a 'performance' (behaving in line with expectations of masculine or feminine behaviour). This approach challenges the conventional view that gender identity is fixed and presents it as socially constructed – a reflection of social expectations (the C level again) rather than biological differences.

Practice focus 7.2

Jim had always assumed that people were born either straight or gay and that people who were gay were in some way an aberration, less than perfect. He did not see himself as a prejudiced individual or in any way discriminatory. He just thought that his beliefs were perfectly natural and normal. However, in the first year of his social work degree he started studying sociology. He learned about how ideologies are sets of powerful ideas that are a key part of how power operates in society. He also learned that what makes an ideology so powerful is that its key ideas become accepted as normal and natural and therefore beyond question and relatively unassailable. He found all this very interesting and stimulating. However, one day the tutor used dominant views about sexuality as an example of how ideology oversimplifies complex ideas and presents dynamic sociopolitical matters as if they were simply fixed biological characteristics. At first he felt very unsettled by this and was resistant to the idea. But, after the group had discussed the issues more fully, he started to think that he would have to look again at some of the things he had been taking for granted.

Paris (2011) discusses the anthropological work of Davies (2007) who writes about the Bugis people from South Sulawesi in Indonesia who conceptualize gender not in binary terms (man/woman), but rather on a continuum across five gender groups as follows:

- men
- calalai (masculine women)
- bissu (transgender shamans)
- calabai (feminine men)
- women

This reinforces the idea, as discussed in Chapter 3, that gender is a social construction rather than a biological given. Different societies at different times in history will have different conceptions of gender. This argument can also be applied to sexuality. We are used to thinking of 'sexual preference' (or sexual orientation) as being a fundamental part of our sense of self or 'identity'. That is, who we are or how we perceive ourselves depends in part on our gender and in part on our sexual orientation. Lawler (2008) argues that sex has come to be seen as not just an activity we engage in, but rather as something that indicates what we *are*. She links this to the work of Foucault, who argued that:

> this way of bringing together sexual desire and identity is fairly recent. It is clear that some people have always engaged in same-sex genital activity, and in some places and times this has been institutionalized (at least between men). But it is only in the late nineteenth century that we see 'the homosexual' appear *as a category of subject*. In this sense, 'homosexuals' (and of course their counterparts, 'heterosexuals') did not exist before the nineteenth century.
>
> (Foucault, 1979, p. 60)

What this indicates is the need to recognize that sexuality is not simply a fixed, biological matter. It is more accurate to see it as a complex multi-dimensional phenomenon (bio-psychosocial and spiritual) which reflects an individual's life experiences over time and the social and historical

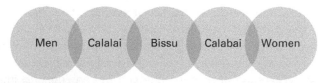

Figure 7.1 Five genders

context in which those experiences have occurred (for an interesting set of discussions about such matters, see Morland and Willox, 2005).

The tendency to see sexuality as fixed is not only theoretically inadequate (because it fails to take account of the wider factors involved), but also problematic at the practice level. This is because the notion of fixed identity is used ideologically to categorize people as either heterosexual (normal/natural/healthy/acceptable/unproblematic) or homosexual (abnormal/unnatural/unhealthy/unacceptable/problematic).

This introduces the concept of 'heteronormativity' (Carabine, 2004a), the idea that sexual diversity is not simply a matter of difference, but rather of *deficit* – a 'pathology'. It is therefore important that, as social workers committed to equality, diversity and social justice, we do not allow the idea of heteronormativity to influence our practice in working with gay, lesbian, bisexual or transsexual people – that is, that we do not unwittingly try to 'normalize' people by expecting them to fit in with heterosexual norms.

If social workers (and, indeed, social work as a professional endeavour more broadly) are to be part of the solution, rather than part of the problem, then we need to be 'tuned in' to issues of sexuality and appreciate their significance in people's lives.

In an earlier work (Thompson, 2015a), I emphasized the importance of self-awareness. Linked to this is the need for social awareness, recognizing how our own personal values and feelings are influenced by our social context and how they, in turn, can influence that social context – especially through our professional practice where we are, in effect, exercising power on behalf of wider society. In this regard, the comments of Canavan and Prior are significant:

> Workers need to be clear about how their personal value base in relation to sexual issues may converge with or diverge from ethical and responsible practice. For example, when it comes to light that a 15-year-old boy is accessing Internet pornography, the worker's own attitude to pornography may affect what is regarded as an appropriate professional response. A male social worker who uses pornography unquestioningly in his private life may minimize the potential harm of this activity to the young person, advocating for the young man's right to privacy, autonomy and freedom of expression, based on an unarticulated assumption that pornography is both ubiquitous and a normal part of male adolescent sexual development. The worker may not be able to undertake the assessment required in this situation to gauge the nature, content, frequency and circumstances of the young person's use of pornography and its consequential impact on his thinking, feelings, attitudes and behaviour.
>
> (Canavan and Prior, 2008, p. 336)

This raises important challenges and reflects an important the͏ cussed elsewhere in this book – the idea that most discrimination is u͏ tentional, based on a lack of awareness and an uncritical acceptance o͏ the dominant ideology (at the **C** level), which reflects and reinforces the deeply ingrained inequalities (at the **S** level), and is not simply a result of direct prejudice and bigotry (at the **P** level).

Canavan and Prior (2008) go on to argue that, as social workers, we have a personal and professional responsibility to work on our own issues around sex, sexual relationships and sexuality if we are to practise responsibly and ethically. They echo my point about the importance of self-awareness and link this to the need to be comfortable with talking openly and explicitly about sex and related matters. If we are not able to get past our own concerns, then we will be in a weak position when it comes to trying to help others.

As a consequence of developing greater self-awareness and social awareness, long-cherished views are likely to be challenged at times. However, the net result of this should be that the social worker will be more responsive to others who are struggling to express any doubts, anxieties or distress in relation to the sexual dimension of their being, and will thus be better equipped to help. They point out the challenging nature of this aspect of social work:

> None of this is easy. It is likely to be fraught and messy at times. It will, however, go a long way towards ensuring that social work clients and social workers themselves are understood and supported in matters relating to their sexuality and sexual relationships.
>
> (Canavan and Prior, 2008, p. 340)

Suitably well-informed and committed social workers can, therefore, make a positive contribution to social justice by offering positive and sensitive help to people who are experiencing difficulties in relation to their sexuality, especially when those difficulties owe much to the discrimination and oppression that heteronormativity in particular and heterosexism in general are sadly characteristic of in contemporary society.

Voice of experience 7.2

Getting past all the prejudice and stereotypes can be difficult, but it's essential that we don't exclude sexuality issues from our anti-oppressive efforts. Even people who seem very enlightened about other aspects of discrimination can be incredibly ill-informed about homophobia. *Gary, a social worker in an intake team*

›ressions

l in earlier chapters, forms of discrimination do not gen- lation – they reflect dimensions of human experience. To develop understanding of heterosexism we therefore need to have at least a basic grasp of how it relates to other forms of discrimination. Space does not permit a comprehensive account of the complexities involved, but the following discussion should at least cast some light on important aspects of the way heterosexism exists alongside – and inter- acts with – other forms of discrimination.

Sanders makes an important point when she argues that:

> So while we have to highlight homophobia, because it's something that people consistently forget, we cannot tackle homophobia on its own. We have to be dealing with racism, sexism, heterosexism, size-ism, you know whatever it is that kids have a go at each other on. That's the thing we actually have to look at. What is in our culture which is constantly enabling and often condoning people treating each other badly?
>
> (Sanders, 2008, p. 7)

Once again, what is presented as applying to children's services can also be extended to apply to social work more broadly defined, regardless of client group.

We can identify clear links between heterosexism and sexism, as both have much to do with identity and established (ideological) expectations about how people should relate to each other in terms of gender roles (sexism) and sexuality/sexual relations (heterosexism). Segal (2007) goes a step further than this in arguing that homophobic persecution, as some- thing that can be seen as generally the actions and attitudes of one group of men against a minority of other men, also involves the 'forced repres- sion of the "feminine" in all men' (2007, p. 13). In this way men are kept separated off from women, which then has the ideological effect of keep- ing women subordinate to men, thereby reinforcing patriarchal power relations. While I feel there are elements of oversimplification in Segal's analysis, her comments help to show that the combination of sexism and heterosexism is not simply a chance coming together of two forms of discrimination from time to time. Rather, they are two interlocking aspects of a complex multidimensional set of power dynamics that play a key part in shaping people's experiences of discrimination (Thompson, 2010).

Heterosexism can also be seen to interrelate with ageism and disablism, in so far as heterosexist attitudes and assumptions can be particularly prob- lematic for older or disabled people, as it is often assumed that they have no sexuality at all, that they are sexless beings. This can be doubly oppressive for older or disabled people whose sexuality does not fit in with heterosexual norms. It is therefore vitally important that social workers should not engage in work with older or disabled people in ways that deny them their sexuality in general or rule out the possibility that their sexual orientation may be anything other than heterosexual.

Practice focus 7.3

Tony had been diagnosed with his illness several years ago, when he was in his early 70s. He knew only too well that his illness was incurable and that he would continue to deteriorate to the extent that, before long, he would be totally dependent on others for every aspect of his physical care. Already he felt bad about relying on Jack, his life partner for more than 25 years, and had come to the decision that the quality of their relationship would be enhanced if he moved to a residential setting where there would be paid carers on hand all of the time. Jack was not at all keen on the idea at first, but felt better after reading the 'Statement of Values' of the home's promotional literature and the reassurance given by the manager that Tony would be treated as a person with his own unique needs.

However, this commitment did not appear to be borne out in practice. Both Tony and Jack had found the transition very traumatic and wanted to spend as much time together as they could. They had always been very demonstrative in their love for each other and found hugging and physical intimacy comforting. Jack would spend at least part of every day with Tony in his room and often lay beside him on the bed embracing him, as had been their usual practice when either of them had felt ill or anxious. While there had been no overt disapproval of their displays of intimacy, they were both very aware of the embarrassed looks on the faces of carers when they entered the room, and they had overheard discussions about how 'weird' it was for people 'of their age' to be behaving in such a manner. And, although they had expected a more enlightened attitude from people working in the caring professions, they were only too aware that it was intimacy between two men, as well as intimacy between two older people that was providing a talking point among the staff.

They had hoped that, as Tony's condition deteriorated, it would be possible for Jack to sleep with him, as those long hours were the time when they both needed the reassurance that physical closeness brought. From their experience so far, they began to doubt whether this would be possible, or even desirable, given the atmosphere it was likely to promote. So much for 'unique needs', thought Jack. After all, they weren't asking for much, surely? Just that they be allowed to comfort each other without being judged according to heterosexist and ageist perceptions of what is 'appropriate'. (S. Thompson, 2005, p. 70)

Towards anti-heterosexist practice

Heterosexism is a deeply ingrained set of ideas and practices both within and outside social work. It is a significant and widespread form of oppression which merits inclusion on the anti-discriminatory practice agenda. Much more work remains to be done to develop a fuller picture of what would be required to develop an adequate basis for anti-heterosexist practice. However, the following points can take us some distance in that direction and help to develop a platform for better theoretical understandings and better-informed practice responses:

1 Identity is an important concept in social work, and so the tendency to neglect issues relating to the sexuality aspects of identity must be resisted. Identity is not something that is fixed (Thompson, 2010) – it is in large part a response to the wider social influences we encounter as we travel through our lives. A social work assessment that neglects such issues is therefore unlikely to be an adequate or acceptable assessment.

Key point 7.2

Identity is a key issue. Undermining, stigmatizing or devaluing a person's identity can have highly detrimental consequences. Such a negative approach to someone's identity is a common by-product of discrimination. We therefore have to be sensitive in relation to people's sense of identity, including their sexual identity.

---

2 In a similar spirit of respecting a person's identity, the 'heterosexual assumption' is something that needs to be avoided. That is, we should not automatically assume that a person is heterosexual, even though the majority of people will be. To make such an assumption has the effect of presenting same-sex relations as deficient, rather than different and therefore pathologizing gay, lesbian or bisexual people. By the same token, we should not make assumptions about people's sexuality based on aspects of appearance or behaviour that may be perceived stereotypically as 'gay'. Sexuality is an important part of a person's sense of self and thus of their spirituality and therefore needs to be treated with respect.

3 We also need to make sure that we do not rely uncritically on dominant understandings of sexual orientation and family life. As Brown and Cocker put it:

> It is important for social workers not to assume that their own experience and knowledge of family forms and structures will or should apply to everyone. It is necessary to hear from lesbian or gay individuals or families how they define the terms 'family' and 'kinship' as meaningful and accurate for themselves. The meaning of family and kinship is not static and will be different for individual clients and carers. ... it will involve acknowledging the importance of bonds of attachment and responsibilities related to care giving towards others that need to be respected and nurtured by social workers wherever possible.
>
> (Brown and Cocker, 2011, p. 77)

4 From an organizational point of view, harassment policies, where they exist, should address harassment on the grounds of sexual orientation or identity (Thompson, 2000b). People can be bullied or harassed for a wide variety of reasons, and it would be naïve and unhelpful not to recognize that sexuality can be a major factor in such problems, leading to considerable distress for the people.

5 Similarly, as Cocker and Hafford-Letchfield (2010) acknowledge, the legal picture relating to sexuality equality has been transformed in recent years by an unprecedented level of new legislation and associated guidance. While it remains the case – as I have argued above – that there is much more to anti-discriminatory practice than legal compliance, there is much to be gained by having a good understanding of the relevant legislation that offers a degree of protection from discrimination on the grounds of sexual orientation.

6 A person's sexual identity should not be seen as a significant factor in terms of risk assessment, eligibility for services and so on. In particular, we need to move away from the simplistic assumption that being gay, lesbian or bisexual is to be equated with being a threat to children. Similarly, we need to make sure that we avoid the common assumption that not being heterosexual is an indicator of possible mental health problems.

7 Training in relation to sexuality and sexual identity should be recognized as a mainstream issue and not marginalized as an issue for specialist workers (HIV counsellors, for example). These are complex issues that need careful consideration, with time for developing theoretical understandings and exploring the implications for practice.

8   It is essential that social workers are comfortable with sexuality issues generally (as highlighted by Canavan and Prior, 2008). If not, then the specific challenges of wrestling with complexities of sexual diversity are likely to be beyond us. We then run the risk of unwittingly contributing to sexuality-based discrimination by giving gay, lesbian or bisexual people a lower level of service than we would do to heterosexual people.

9   We should not put pressure on people to 'come out' if they choose not to, but if they do, then we should be prepared to give them appropriate support, as it needs to be recognized that the anxieties and pressures involved can be quite significant.

10 Although there has been much progress in moving away from overt disapproval of same-sex relations, discriminatory comments, attitudes and behaviours continue to be a feature of social life. It is therefore important that we are able to challenge – sensitively, skilfully and constructively (see the discussion of 'elegant challenging' in *Promoting Equality*) – any such manifestations of heterosexism.

Food for thought

● How might your own experiences of sexuality colour the way you practise as a social worker?

● Can you identify stereotypes of gay, lesbian or bisexual people? How can you ensure that your practice does not rely on such stereotypical assumptions?

● In what ways might a person's sexuality affect the needs they have and the problems they encounter?

Further resources

Canavan and Prior ('Sexuality and Sexual Relationships', 2008) is a useful starting point for a discussion of sexuality in relation to social work. Brown and Cocker (*Social Work with Lesbians and Gay Men*, 2011) provides a more detailed, extended analysis of some of the key issues discussed in this chapter. The Equality and Human Rights Commission Report (*Beyond Tolerance: Making Sexual Orientation a Public Matter*, 2009) provides a useful overview of the need for equality measures.
Morland and Willox (*Queer Theory*, 2005) is an interesting and thought-provoking set of readings about queer theory. Carabine (*Sexualities: Personal Lives and*

Social Policy, 2004b) is also a useful set of readings, but with a policy emphasis rather than a theoretical one. DePalma and Atkinson (*Invisible Boundaries: Addressing Sexualities Equality in Children's Worlds*, 2008) provide a range of interesting chapters that concentrate on how sexual equalities issues can be addressed in work with children and young people.

Simpson (*Middle-Aged Men, Ageing and Ageism: Over the Rainbow?*, 2015) explores links between heterosexism and ageism. Clarke et al. (*Lesbian, Gay, Bisexual, Trans and Queer Psychology: An Introduction*, 2010) address sexuality issues from a psychological perspective, while Moon (*Feeling Queer or Queer Feelings? Radical Approaches to Counselling, Sex, Sexualities and Genders*, 2008) explores counselling issues.

CHAPTER 8

FAITH AND RELIGIOUS DISCRIMINATION

CHAPTER OVERVIEW

In this chapter you will:

- Learn about how discrimination can arise on the basis of membership of a religious group (and in some cases on the basis of having no religion)
- Explore how political events in recent years have fuelled religious discrimination against Muslims (what has come to be referred to as 'Islamophobia')
- Consider the implications of religious discrimination for professional practice

Introduction

Religion is, of course, a major social institution that has profound effects on social organization, politics, the economy, cultural norms and, not least, personal beliefs and values. The potency of religion is therefore immense.

The term 'religion' is frequently used in the singular as if it were a single, unified concept or force. However, we should not allow this to distract us from recognizing the plurality of religions, the fact that we live in a multi-faith society. There exists a multiplicity of religions and, within the major religions, a number of 'subdivisions' or variations as, for example, in the Islamic faith. Such religious diversity is often closely linked with ethnic or racial groupings, although not exclusively so. Indeed, a sensitivity to, and awareness of, religious values and practices is a significant component of ethnically sensitive practice as discussed in Chapter 4.

Unfortunately I have come across many people who make the mistake of assuming that modern society is predominantly secular and that religion is therefore a relatively minor consideration. Holloway and Moss (2010) point out that, in the 2001 census in England and Wales, only 15 per cent of people claimed to have no religious affiliation. To ignore religion and its significance in social work is therefore a significant mistake. Similarly, to ignore religious discrimination is potentially very problematic.

To begin to develop an understanding of religious discrimination, we can recognize that religion can be seen to be significant in relation to all three levels of PCS analysis:

P – religious beliefs are a fundamental part of many people's identity and can therefore be a major guide to action on the basis of moral principles or required practices (for example, rituals). For a high proportion of people their sense of who they are and how they fit into the wider world is largely a matter of their religion. Their religion colours all aspects of their lives and their relationships with other people and wider society.

C – shared cultural norms and values often owe much to religion and can be enshrined in the particular religion's system of symbolic representations of reality. Indeed, this is a major feature of religion as a social and existential phenomenon: its ability to bring people together with a strong sense of being united in common cause and common endeavour (the flipside of this, as Moss, 2005, perceptively acknowledges, is that a strong sense of adherence to one faith group can lead to conflict with other faith groups – we shall return to this point below).

S – stratification systems can be based on religion (for example, caste) and, indeed, the links between religion and wider sociopolitical factors have been extensively explored (for example, Weber's study, *The Protestant Ethic and the Spirit of Capitalism*, first published in 1904).

Religion can play a central part in the lives of social work clients at a number of levels and therefore needs to be taken into account in social work assessment, intervention, evaluation and policy planning (Moss, 2005; Holloway and Moss, 2010). This needs to be part of the broader recognition that everyone has spiritual needs, everyone faces the existential challenges of finding or creating threads of meaning that help us make sense of our lives. This in turn needs to be seen as part of social work (and, arguably, the helping professions in general), in so far as helping people to develop new more empowering meanings or 'narratives' has an important part to play in the social worker's repertoire (Thompson, 2010). For very many people those spiritual needs will be met, in part at least, through religion. To discriminate against someone because of their religion can therefore amount to striking at the very heart of their being, potentially doing considerable damage to self-esteem, personal security and thus to overall well-being. Consequently, the potential for religious discrimination (including unwitting discrimination) is something we need to be aware of and be prepared to address.

What is religious discrimination?

Having clarified, to some extent, the need to take account of religious factors in general and the question of religious discrimination in particular, let us now turn our attention to developing a clearer picture of what is involved.

At its simplest, religious discrimination is, as the term implies, discrimination against individuals or groups on the basis of their faith or religious beliefs. However, we need to recognize that there are variations on this theme. Consider the following:

- Discrimination by members of one religion against another – for example, Sikhs being made to feel that they are not welcome in a predominantly Christian organization.

- Discrimination by members of one sect (that is, subsection of a religion) against another within the same overall religion. Sectarianism involving Catholics and Protestants would be a clear example of this.

- Members of one particular subsection of a religious group being discriminated against because they are deemed to be less worthy than others – for example, the 'dalits' (or 'untouchables' as they were previously known) within the caste system associated with Hinduism.

- Non-religious people discriminating against people of any religion (that is, being anti-religious as well as non-religious) – for example, people's religious beliefs and rituals being dismissed as 'hokum' or 'mumbo-jumbo'.

- Religious people discriminating against non-believers, dismissing them as 'godless' – for example, some members of a religious organization trying to block the employment of non-religious people within that organization.

It is also important to recognize that religious discrimination can be categorized as either intentional (based on prejudice at the **P** level, perhaps reinforced by stereotypes and distorted representations at the **C** level and economic or other interests at the **S** level) or unintentional (based on institutionalized assumptions and patterns of behaviour that have developed over time as a result of influences from the **C** and **S** levels). I shall return to this distinction below, as it is important that we are aware of both types of discriminatory processes.

al injury and was undergoing a process of rehabilitation. Mrs
ry of depression and, since her husband's accident, had
pressed. They had two young children and the GP's concern
needed a lot of support at the moment to ensure that the
ared for in difficult circumstances. Siobhan had written to Mr
and Mrs ~~~~~~ arrange an appointment and had signed the letter, S. Davies
(her married name). When she arrived at the house Mr Carlton seemed very wel-
coming but, once she introduced herself as Siobhan Davies, Mr Carlton became
quite cold towards her and seemed reluctant to talk to her. He had a northern
English accent but she could detect traces of a Northern Ireland accent. She
later found out that he was from a Protestant family that had moved to England
after Mr Carlton's brother had been killed in a bomb explosion during the Troubles. Siobhan wondered whether her name, traditionally seen as an Irish Catholic
name, was the reason for Mr Carlton suddenly turning cold towards her.

Islamophobia

Of course, sectarianism is not the only example of the interaction of religion and oppression or discrimination. Religion is a highly significant
dimension of our existence at a number of levels and a wide variety of
examples could be given of problems arising from conflicting religious
ideologies and related matters. One such example which has received
considerable attention in recent years is the development and intensifica-
tion of negative attitudes and actions towards Muslims. Since the terrorist
attacks of 9/11 (that is, the attacks on the World Trade Center in New York
and the Pentagon US military headquarters on the 11th of September,
2001) and subsequent attacks attributed to, or claimed by, Al-Qaeda, for
many people in the west there is now a strong association between terrorism and Islam. This is an unfair and misleading distortion of reality, but
unfortunately we now have a situation in which there are serious and
significant tensions in the United States, the United Kingdom and other
Anglophone countries in relation to Muslims.

Key point 8.1

Discrimination is often reinforced by (misguided) public opinion and/or distorted media representations. We need to make sure that our practice is based
on our professional knowledge base about such matters and not on popular
opinion, however strongly or frequently that opinion might be expressed.

There is a considerable irony here, as Islam is a religion based on peace (in fact, the name 'Islam' means 'peace' or 'way to peace'). While there are clearly some Muslims who are engaged in terrorist activities, this recognition is, of course, a far cry from assuming that Islam is a religion that stands for terrorism or that Muslims in general engage in or support terrorism. Despite this, we have none the less seen a considerable growth in antipathy towards people of Muslim faith, a growth in terms of what has come to be known as 'Islamophobia' (fear or hatred of Islam as a religion and Muslims as people). Gilliat-Ray (2010) points out that Muslim identity has come to be distorted. She argues that:

> The trouble with this is that Muslims cannot be seen simply as human beings: they have to be perceived mainly through the religious prism. Giving them a one-dimensional description, however important, undervalues the complexity of that person (Hussain, D. 2008: 40).
>
> (Gilliat-Ray, 2010, p. xi)

An important report prepared by the Runnymede Trust and published in 1997 identified eight characteristics associated with Islamophobia:

1 Islam is seen as a monolithic bloc, static and unresponsive to change.

2 Islam is seen as separate and 'other'. It does not have values in common with other cultures, is not affected by them and does not influence them.

3 Islam is seen as inferior to the West. It is seen as barbaric, irrational, primitive and sexist.

4 Islam is seen as violent, aggressive, threatening, supportive of terrorism and engaged in a 'clash of civilizations'.

5 Islam is seen as a political ideology and is used for political or military advantage.

6 Criticisms made of the West by Islam are rejected out of hand.

7 Hostility towards Islam is used to justify discriminatory practices towards Muslims and exclusion of Muslims from mainstream society.

8 Anti-Muslim hostility is seen as natural or normal.

(www.islamophobia-watch.com/islamophobia-a-definition)

These eight features illustrate the workings of ideology at the **C** level which both influences actions and attitudes at the **P** level and reflects social divisions at the **S** level. It shows how distorted, misleading and unfair such cultural assumptions can be and how they can encourage conflict and hostility. It is therefore essential that social workers are not influenced by such unhelpful and discriminatory assumptions, that we are able to distance ourselves from the stereotypical perceptions that feed discrimination against Muslims.

The implications for social work

There are various ways in which we can try to ensure that, when it comes to religious discrimination, we are part of the solution and not part of the problem. I shall highlight some of these here, although it needs to be recognized that my comments are far from comprehensive or exhaustive – they represent just a selection of important issues. We are still very much at the beginning of developing our understanding of religious discrimination, and indeed our understanding of the significance of spiritual matters in general as they relate to social work (Holloway and Moss, 2010).

One very simple but none the less important consideration to be aware of is that social work records will often require the worker to indicate someone's religion. Unfortunately, for many workers this can simply mean ticking a box on a form (or computer screen) without giving any thought to what a person's religion means to them. For some people their religion plays only a minor role in their lives, whereas for others, their religion is a central part of who they are, how they live their lives and how they relate to other people. We should therefore remember that, when it comes to identifying someone's religion, it is more than a matter of ticking a box.

The logic of this can also be applied to assessment more broadly. An assessment should involve gathering relevant information to form a picture of the situation so that a plan for what needs to be done can be developed. In many cases religious factors will be major features of that picture, and so to omit them would present a very partial and distorted understanding on which to base our plans and intervention. Of course, it will not always be the case that religion is a significant part of the story, but if we assume that it is not without exploring the possibility, then we are practising dangerously.

One thing that would make this dangerous practice is that we would be contributing to discrimination by neglecting key aspects of an individual's or family's religious affiliation and identity. We would be giving them a lower level of service and professional practice than we would to people for whom religion has no particular significance, and that would therefore constitute discrimination. We should note, though, that even in working with people who express no religious affiliation, their spirituality will still be a key factor to take into consideration.

A further important point to bear in mind is that we need to be aware of the possible impact of discrimination in people's lives that may otherwise not feature in our thinking. Just as it would be poor practice to work with, say, a black family and not consider racism as part of the presenting situation, it would be a serious mistake to work with a family who are committed to a particular religion without also exploring whether they have experienced, are experiencing or are worried about experiencing discrimination on the grounds of their religion. Of course, we should not assume automatically that such a family or individuals within it are encountering discrimination, but nor should we rule out the possibility. We could be denying people the opportunity to explore ways of countering the discrimination that features in their lives (and which may be exacerbating other problems in their lives).

Last but not least, for present purposes, is the question of access to faith community resources. Unfortunately I have come across many cases of social workers adopting a very narrow perspective and drawing on a very limited range of helping options. This can often include not taking account of the possibility of resources being available through an individual's or family's faith community. Very often religious groups are able to provide practical and emotional support for members of their church (and sometimes for non-members too). A narrow, unimaginative response to people's needs may result in their losing out in terms of potential sources of help which could have the added bonus of helping them connect more fully with their faith community.

The anti-discriminatory response

There have been a variety of responses to religious discrimination, legal, political and professional. It is beyond the scope of this book to provide a detailed discussion of current and historical legal provision, as it is quite complex.

In a nutshell, the Human Rights Act 1998 offers some degree of protection. According to Article 9 of the European Convention on Human Rights:

1 Everyone has the right to freedom of thought, conscience and religion; this right includes freedom to change his [sic] religion or belief and freedom, either alone or in community with others and in public or private, to manifest his religion or belief, in worship, teaching, practice and observance.

2 Freedom to manifest one's religion or beliefs shall be subject only to such limitations as are prescribed by law and are necessary in a democratic society in the interests of public safety, for the protection of public order, health or morals, or for the protection of the rights and freedoms of others.

The implementation of the Equality Act 2010 introduced the idea of 'protected characteristics', and religion or belief is one of them (alongside age, disability, gender reassignment, marriage and civil partnership, pregnancy or maternity, race, sex and sexual orientation). This means that there is some protection from discrimination on the grounds of religion. While the legal framework is not comprehensive, it does give us a foundation of legal protection on which to build a commitment to equality.

In terms of political responses, we have seen major anti-sectarian initiatives through the peace process in Northern Ireland and smaller initiatives elsewhere (for example, efforts to rid football of sectarianism in Scotland). In relation to Islam, we can see efforts to promote equality through such movements as Islamophobia Watch (www.islamophobia-watch.com). The Runnymede Trust, through its development and publication of the report, *Islamophobia: A Challenge for Us All* (1997) has also made an important contribution. In addition, the Commission on British Muslims and Islamophobia has produced an important report, *Islamophobia: Issues, Challenges and Action* (2004). While we still have a long way to go yet, we can see that there is a foundation of political resistance to religious discrimination.

From a professional point of view, we can see that there has been a growing awareness of the need to incorporate religious issues into social work and the helping professions more broadly (see, for example, Furness and Gilligan, 2009). This can be seen as a growing awareness of the significance of spirituality in people's lives (Holloway and Moss, 2010;

Moss, 2005). This development, I would argue, also owes much to the development of the diversity approach, which includes, of course, religious and spiritual diversity. Moss provides an important perspective when he argues that:

> One of the litmus tests of a civilized society is the way in which minority groups are regarded and treated by the majority. This involves the extent to which people who belong to minority groups are marginalized or victimized. We would want to argue that a truly mature society is not marked out so much by its tolerance of difference, important though that undoubtedly is, but the extent to which it positively celebrates difference, and cherishes and encourages it as an enrichment.

> Events around the world and in the UK in recent years have demonstrated just how perilous and important such a vision for society has become. In moments of tension or attack, some of the tolerance and acceptance of various groups in society can quickly dissolve. Groups can be targeted and scapegoated, and the cherished principles of a multicultural community (however that is to be defined) are put at risk.
>
> (Moss, 2007, p. 46)

He goes on to make the equally important point that this is a matter of values. I would therefore want to emphasize that a commitment to tackling religious discrimination needs to be based on professional values and not simply compliance with legal requirements.

In addition, while it would be a mistake to see religious discrimination as simply an element of racism (see the discussion below), the sustained efforts to challenge racism over the decades has also gone some way to challenging at least some aspects of discrimination based on religion.

Voice of experience 8.2

So many people have assumed over the years that because I am male, heterosexual, not disabled and I don't have black or brown skin, I can't have experienced discrimination. But, believe me, when your name is Cohen, you don't have to wait long before you get the discriminatory stereotypes left, right and centre.
Amos, a child protection social worker

Multiple oppressions

Religions provide sets of symbols and an overall worldview which offers their adherents a means of making sense of the world. In this way, religion provides a basis for understanding other social divisions (for example, how older or disabled people are perceived and treated – they may be respected and revered as 'elders' in such religions as Jainism and Hinduism, rather than demeaned and marginalized as 'the elderly'). There are therefore likely to be significant linkages across the different forms of discrimination, with complex dynamics of interaction taking place.

In particular, we can recognize that there are close links with racism. This is because part of racism is a fear and rejection of what is seen as foreign or alien (the exact opposite of valuing diversity), and this is also a key feature of religious discrimination, in so far as people brought up in one faith (or in no faith at all) can find the rituals, symbolism and iconography, language, beliefs and behaviour associated with another creed quite alien and unfamiliar (this is part of what Bauman, 2000, calls 'heterophobia' – fear of what is different). Without a value commitment to equality and diversity, such feelings can play a part in fuelling discriminatory sentiments and actions. These, in turn, can be specifically religious (that is, directed specifically at a person's religious beliefs and/or identity), more broadly racist (directed more generally at people who are perceived to be part of a particular 'race' or ethnic group) or a combination of the two.

Practice focus 8.2

Mohamed was a team manager in a drugs and alcohol team. Throughout his life he had unfortunately encountered racism many times, in both his personal and professional life. It was not uncommon, for example, for clients who were under the effects of alcohol or other drugs to be racially abusive towards him. However, after the Al-Qaeda terrorist attacks in central London, he noticed that there was a switch in the nature of the abuse. Now he found that the venom was directed at him as a Muslim and he was told on more than one occasion that he was a 'no-good Muslim terrorist who should go back home'. He found it interesting to note that he was still receiving as much negativity as usual, but now for a different reason.

However, in considering religious discrimination and racism, it is important that we do not conflate the two and thereby miss the differences between them. For example, the Commission on British Muslims and Islamophobia (2004) points out that a third of Britis| Asian and half of all Asians are not Muslims. So, while ι significant overlap between Islam and perceived racial g are also significant differences. In working with people w religious and an ethnic minority, we therefore have to look ﹍ ﹍ the situation to see whether any discrimination involved in the situation is specifically religious, specifically racist or both.

Class issues can also interact with religious discrimination, in so far as religious communities can cut across class boundaries, but are often in line with them. For example, the Commission on British Muslims and Islamophobia (2004) points out that Muslims in Britain are disproportionately affected by poverty and social exclusion. We therefore need to be aware of the interactions of class and religious factors and how, for example, they may exacerbate each other.

We also need to consider language discrimination, as discussed in Chapter 1, as this too can interact in significant ways with religion. The use of a particular language can be a marker of cultural, national or religious identity and can also, at times, amount to making a strong political statement. Language, then is a complex sociopolitical phenomenon (Joseph, 2004; Millar, 2005) and can be linked with discrimination in a number of ways – for example, someone speaking Irish becoming the victim of sectarian discrimination. By the same token, someone who has anti-semitic beliefs may not realize that a particular person is Jewish (and therefore show no animosity towards them), but may change their approach to that person when they realize, say, that the newspaper they are reading is written in Yiddish or Hebrew. Language discrimination can therefore combine with religious discrimination in complex and subtle ways.

The example of sectarianism is a helpful one for understanding how different forms of discrimination interact and reinforce each other. In particular, anti-sectarianism has now come to be seen as part of a broader project of tackling discrimination and oppression. Heenan and Birrell comment that:

> Sectarianism in Northern Ireland can be seen as demonstrating a close relationship with other forms of prejudice on the basis of race, gender or disability, and thus anti-sectarian practice can be linked to anti-discriminatory practice and compared to such measures in Britain. Consequently, Northern Ireland practice can be examined for any particular insights that might be applicable in Great Britain. This is more relevant with the high profile now given to issues of religious identity

discrimination on religious grounds in Great Britain. The absorption of anti-sectarianism into broader equality provision and good relations duties has provided a means of resolving the potential conflict between radical discourses of anti-oppressive practice and values, and more conservative and regulatory forms of social work practice.

(Heenan and Birrell, 2011, p. 36)

There is a parallel here with the Welsh context. At one time campaigns for promoting the Welsh language and culture and protecting them from discriminatory assumptions that they have no role in a globalizing world had little connection with wider political movements committed to equality and diversity. However, matters relating to Welsh language and culture are now firmly part of the broader professional and political agenda of promoting equality and challenging discrimination and oppression. For example, the Welsh internationalist political party, Plaid Cymru, now has a clear and firm commitment to social justice in general and not just in relation to language and culture.

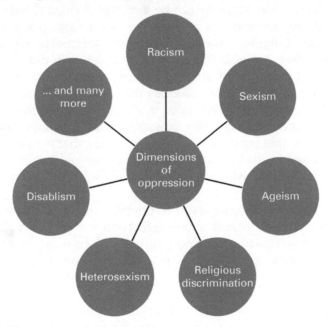

Figure 8.1 Dimensions of oppression

A further example of the interaction of different forms of discrimination is the restriction on women and the resulting gender inequalities enshrined in some religious doctrines. A commonly quoted example of this is the status of women in Islam and the apparent assignment of them to a secondary position. However, this is a complex matter, and we should be careful not to oversimplify. For example, Shah (2006) argues that the Koran is supportive of women's status and that it is how this holy book is interpreted in particular Muslim states at particular times in history that produces the tendency to assign women to subordinate roles (see also Vatuk, 2008). As with sectarianism, then, we can have what appear to be fundamentally religious issues which, on closer inspection, can be seen as part of a much broader, multidimensional social context in which power dynamics are operating at different levels. It is therefore important to recognize that gender factors and religious issues are likely to interact in ways that are significant in both general terms and more specifically in relation to discrimination. However, we must be careful not to oversimplify complex issues.

There is also the thorny matter of religion and heterosexism. Some religions – Christianity, for example – are characterized by an apparent rejection of sexuality equality, and there can be no doubt that many proponents of this and other religions openly reject the validity of gay, lesbian or bisexual identities and associated rights. However, Paris (2011), writing from an overtly Christian perspective, presents a persuasive argument that the Church can accommodate sexual diversity without compromising its principles or tenets. Once again, we need to be careful not to oversimplify complex situations – for example, by assuming that a Christian will automatically be anti-gay. We have to recognize that religion is one social division among many and, as I have argued earlier in this book and elsewhere (*Promoting Equality*, for example), we need to be tuned in to how such divisions (and the forms of discrimination associated with them) interact in complex and changing ways.

Practice focus 8.3

Sandy needed to develop a list of the religions practised within the catchment area of the office where she was on placement. This was to be partly a learning exercise for herself and partly to develop a useful resource for the team. She was able to find out a great deal from the Internet, but she also wanted to meet people from the different religions to get a better feel for what the particular faith was all about. She realized that she had limited time for the project so she pressed on as quickly as she could and was delighted that all the faith leaders she contacted were pleased to welcome her. As she went about her business meeting each faith leader, Sandy became fascinated by what she learned. When the people she met with realized that she was a social work student they started talking to her about the social problems their communities faced. Sandy had a strong interest in anti-discriminatory practice, and so she was able to see how various forms of discrimination were affecting various members of the communities she visited. When she discussed this with her practice teacher, he commented that, on top of the ageism, disablism and so on that she had been hearing about, for many of the people concerned, there would also be religious discrimination to add to their pressures. This project and her practice teacher's comments on it had really hammered home to her that she needed to think about discrimination in a holistic and dynamic way and not reduce it to different 'isms' operating in isolation. She had also learned that, for many people, religious discrimination is part of this complex whole too.

Towards anti-discriminatory practice

This is a vast and complex area and I have only barely begun to scratch the surface in my treatment of the issues here. Much work remains to be done before our understanding of these matters even begins to approach a level of adequacy (although Moss, 2005, is a good step in the right direction). It is important that social workers acknowledge the complexity and vastness of this dimension of social interaction and thus recognize the need to seek advice and guidance in dealing with such issues.

Key point 8.2

While religion arguably features less in people's lives than was the case for earlier generations, it is a mistake of major proportions to neglect the role of religion in general in people's lives and the role of religious discrimination in particular.

It is not possible for social workers to be 'experts' in this area, given our current level of knowledge. None the less, this should not be used as an excuse for failing to address such issues to the best of our abilities. It is through making such attempts that much of the necessary learning will take place. While it would be unrealistic to expect social work staff to have the necessary knowledge of the variety of religions they are likely to encounter, it is quite realistic to expect the appropriate literature to be consulted as and when required (see, the 'Further resources' section at the end of the chapter).

1 We need to be aware that religious discrimination is a feature of many people's lives and merits close attention, just like any other form of discrimination. We have to be careful to avoid the trap of failing to consider religion as a possible source of discrimination. There is a danger that we could miss significant aspects of a person's life and therefore be basing our work on a far from adequate assessment.

2 We also need to recognize that religious discrimination is not simply an aspect or by-product of racism. Racism and religious discrimination can operate together in subtle and complex ways, but they can also arise independently of one another. As is the case with discrimination generally, we need to look carefully at how different social forces interact and not simply adopt a static, one-dimensional view of the situation.

3 But ethnically sensitive practice does need to take account of religious matters. You are not expected to be an expert in the world's religions, but it is clearly important to know at least the basics of a particular religion in working with an individual or family from a faith group that we are not familiar with and be prepared to find out more as needed. Of course, if we are working effectively in partnership with our clients, then we should be able to learn a great deal about the significance of religion directly from them, although we should not make the mistake of expecting them to occupy a teacher role for our benefit.

4 Be aware that a person's religion is likely to influence their identity and their outlook on the world – this may be very different from your own and may therefore be potentially challenging in some ways. Sometimes it will be very clear how someone's worldview reflects their religion, but often it will not. We need to remember that members of a particular religion are not just puppets who all follow their faith's teachings to the letter. There will be considerable variations in how people interpret their religion's expectations of them and in how devout they are.

5 Be aware of your own views about religion and your own sense of spirituality, as these are likely to influence how you approach other people's religious and spiritual perspectives. Regardless of whether you have strong and explicit

/s on such matters or have barely given them any thought, it is
...₃ɪly likely that they will colour how you see the world in general
and those aspects of the world you encounter in your work in
particular.

6 Be prepared to talk openly about differences of perspective. Effective
working relationships need to be based on trust and mutual understanding. Therefore, if there are any differences between your own
perspective and that of the people you are working with, it may be
necessary and helpful to talk about these constructively in a spirit of
developing good partnership working.

7 Do not make assumptions about how people practise their religion –
there are likely to be many variations. For example, many people will
attend their church or place of worship regularly; others may go only
occasionally, while others may never attend, but would still regard
themselves as members of that religion. Similarly, not all Catholics
refrain from practising birth control. Making such assumptions could
give us a distorted picture of the situation we are dealing with.

8 Be aware of the strengths of faith communities and the potential
resources available. It is a very easy mistake for busy practitioners to
make to think narrowly in terms of a limited range of problem-solving
and support options and not think in terms of the potential help that
could be called upon from within their faith community. Conversely,
we should not assume that members of a religious group will not
need additional resources because 'they look after their own', and
nor should we assume that a member of a faith community will want
or welcome support from within that community. There is, of course,
no substitute for a proper assessment.

9 Be prepared to challenge religious discrimination when you encounter it. Whether the discrimination is based on individual acts or institutionalized in social and organizational patterns, intentional or
unintentional, failing to challenge it amounts to condoning it. The
only exception should be the very rare possible situation in which to
challenge such discrimination may place ourselves or other people at
risk of violence or other harm.

10 Seek advice and guidance when and where you need it. Religion is a
complex matter, especially when we consider the multiplicity of faith
groups and the multidimensional interactions across different social
divisions (including religion). Religious discrimination is perhaps

equally complex and, while we have decades of knowledge to draw upon in terms of our understanding of such forms of discrimination as racism and sexism, we are still in the early stages of building up knowledge of religious discrimination (for example, there is relatively little research available). We should not therefore have any qualms about asking for advice and guidance where we need it.

Food for thought

- How would you identify yourself in terms of religion or your spiritual worldview? How might this influence your practice?
- In what ways might religious discrimination feature in the type of work you undertake?
- Whose help might you seek to deal with religious discrimination issues?
- What harm do you think might be done by taking no account of people's religious or spiritual identity or affiliation?

Further resources

Two good texts about religion and spirituality as they apply to social work are Moss (*Religion and Spirituality*, 2005) and Holloway and Moss (*Spirituality and Social Work*, 2010). Moss (2005) has a guide to further learning section that offers useful guidance on relevant websites. For a discussion of sectarianism, see Heenan and Birrell (*Social Work in Northern Ireland: Conflict and Change*, 2011). A very good source relating to Islamophobia is the report produced by the Commission on British Muslims and Islamophobia (*Islamophobia: Issues, Challenges and Action*, 2004). Also of interest are Green (*Fear of Islam: An Introduction to Islamophobia in the West*, 2015) and Kundnani (*The Muslims are Coming!: Islamophobia, Extremism and the Domestic War on Terror*, 2015).
A useful short introduction to Islam is provided by Kaltner (*Islam: What Non-Muslims Should Know*, 2003). Smart (*The World's Religions*, 1998) is a classic and well-loved introduction to world religions and there are very many texts that provide short introductions to various religions.
Gilleat-Ray (*Muslims in Britain: An Introduction*, 2010) offers an interesting historical perspective that challenges a number of modern assumptions.

CHAPTER 9

CONCLUSION

CHAPTER OVERVIEW

In this chapter you will:

- By way of conclusion, be reminded of the main themes on which the book is based
- Recognize the important steps that need to be taken to take anti-discriminatory practice forward
- Consider some of the main pitfalls to be avoided in developing genuinely anti-discriminatory practice

Introduction

Establishing a basis of equality, diversity and social justice in social work is no easy matter. The situation is made extremely complex by virtue of the number of forms of discrimination, the subtle and intricate ways they manifest themselves and the vested power interests which act as obstacles to change. Consequently, there can be no simple formula solutions which give a clear and straightforward path to follow.

The full development of anti-discriminatory practice must be a longer-term aim if more than lip service is to be achieved. This does not mean that significant improvements and advances cannot be made in the short term. Indeed, the establishment of a strong edifice of anti-discriminatory policy and practice in the long term will depend on the firm foundations to be laid in the short term. The success of such a venture must depend ultimately on collective action and commitment. But each individual has a part to play in the major change from traditional approaches to social work to a form of practice based on principles of emancipatory practice – countering the various forms and processes of discrimination and the oppression they produce.

This book is intended as a guide for those who wish to play their part in this major change. But it must be recognized that it is only a guide; in itself it cannot produce emancipatory practice. It can only make a contribution by:

- helping to develop the necessary knowledge base;
- stimulating debate, discussion and further study of the relevant issues;
- motivating readers to develop the skills, values and attitudes needed;
- encouraging the creation of support groups and a collective approach; and
- acting as an introduction, and bridge, to other more specialist texts on the subject.

If the book is to play a significant part in helping to promote genuine anti-discriminatory practice it is important that its key messages are not lost or diverted. It is therefore regrettable that some people have misrepresented my work as represented in earlier editions of this book. It is important to note, for example, that Dominelli (2002) is incorrect to suggest that my work promotes an idea of a hierarchy of oppressions (that is, the idea that some forms of discrimination are more important than others). I have never supported such an idea and have explicitly stated on more than one occasion that forms of discrimination are dimensions of people's experience and have to be understood holistically, hence the discussion in previous editions of this book – and the present edition – of the importance of understanding how different forms of discrimination interact with one another. That is far removed from what Dominelli calls an 'additive' approach.

Laird is also incorrect to suggest that the way I present race is essentialist. I certainly do not 'essentialize "black" and "white", ascribing to them fixed characteristics normally associated with "race"' (2008, p. 24). All my published work has been rooted in existentialism (Thompson, 1992; 2010; 2012), a key feature of which is a rejection of essentialism. No careful or fair reading of my work could conclude that I 'essentialize white people, slotting them into the same category without differentiation' (Laird, 2008, p. 27). The discussion – in all five editions of this book – of Welsh language issues is just one example among many of the recognition that white people are not a homogeneous group. I would also like to point out quite emphatically that, despite what Laird states, I do not believe that white people are by definition racist – in fact, the prevalence of such simplistic and reductionist ideas was one of the primary motivations for my writing the first edition of this book. The development of PCS analysis was intended to illustrate the complexities of discrimination and the dangers of adopting an oversimplified, essentialist view of very intricate and constantly changing matters. This rejection of essentialism and reductionism is further discussed in both Thompson (2009b) and in *Promoting Equality*.

It is disappointing to note that Bhatti-Sinclair also misrepresents my work. She cites the fourth edition of this book as an example of an approach to discrimination and oppression that 'steers change and development through the application of law' (2011, p. 69), even though that edition, like this one, explicitly stated that it is a mistake to restrict anti-discriminatory practice to matters of law. She is also wrong to suggest that my work reflects the idea that 'BME individuals and communities ... require structures which enable unification and conformity' (2011, p. 69). That is certainly not an idea I would support and not one that features in my work. It is therefore important for me to distance myself from these distortions and misrepresentations of my work. These are classic examples of a polemical approach: falsely attribute a view or analysis to someone and then criticize that person for subscribing to a view that they do not hold or an analysis they have not put forward! Such poor scholarship hinders rather than helps the development of emancipatory forms of practice.

To facilitate meeting the book's aims it would be helpful to restate some of the main themes, by way of a concluding summary, and to examine some of the issues affecting the way forward.

The main themes

There have been a number of recurring themes and it is perhaps worth commenting on seven of these in particular:

Power

Social work is a political activity – that is, it operates within the context of sets of power relations: the power of law and the state, the power inherent in social divisions such as class, race and gender, and the micro-level power of personal interactions. Indeed, power can be seen to operate at all three levels, personal, cultural and structural (Thompson, 2007; 2011a). Also, many of the problems social workers tackle have their roots in the abuse of power – child abuse, for example.

Diversity

We live and work in a society characterized by considerable diversity. Difference is therefore a key issue. It is important that we recognize the danger of (perceptions of) difference becoming the basis of unfair discrimination and thus oppression. Diversity and difference can be seen as assets to be valued and celebrated – sources of stimulation and enrichment, rather than problems to be solved.

PCS analysis

Traditional social work relates primarily to the level of the individual, with only limited recognition of the level of culture, values and shared meanings. Anti-discriminatory practice, by contrast, takes a much wider view – indeed a holistic perspective – which takes account of all three levels – **P**, **C** and **S** – and the interactions between them. It is not sufficient to address only the **P** level (as in many traditional forms of practice) or only the structural (as in the less sophisticated versions of radical social work) – an analysis that does justice to the complexities of social work must have a broader focus, encompassing a range of issues at all three levels.

Ideology

An ideology is a set of ideas which both reflects and reinforces a set of power relations with which it is associated. For example, patriarchal ideology both reflects the powerful position of men in relation to women and, by promoting sexism, reinforces that power. Ideology acts as the 'glue' which binds together the three levels of PCS analysis and, as such, has considerable discriminatory potential.

Oppression

Certain actions, attitudes and structures have the effect of oppressing particular individuals and groups – specifically those 'out groups' that are discriminated against within the social structure (subaltern groups, to use the technical term). Often oppression is unintended on the part of individuals, but none the less deeply ingrained in cultural patterns and institutional structures. Unfair discrimination is the primary source of oppression.

Empowerment

Traditional approaches to social work take little or no account of the oppression inherent in certain aspects of social organization. They therefore see the social work task as one of adjustment to the 'natural order of things', rather than a contribution to the political struggle against oppression. Thus, the focus in anti-discriminatory practice is on empowerment rather than adjustment, challenging injustice rather than simply accepting it as inevitable.

No middle road

Social work practice cannot avoid the question of discrimination and oppression. The actions of social workers and the policies of their agencies will have the effect of either: (a) challenging and undermining, on a minor scale at least, the discrimination to which clients are subject; or (b) tacitly condoning and thus reinforcing such discrimination. There can be no middle road.

There are, of course, many other themes and issues which have arisen, but it is to be hoped that the seven outlined above encapsulate the main thrust of the philosophy of emancipatory practice expounded here. But how can these themes be integrated into day-to-day practice? How can they become an established part of social work? These are some of the issues I now wish to explore, in outline at least, and to focus on some of the dangers and obstacles which can stand in the way of developing a firm foundation of anti-discriminatory practice.

The way forward

Chapters 3 to 8 each ended with some guidance and suggestions concerning the implementation of principles of anti-discriminatory practice in relation to the particular area of discrimination being discussed. It is to be hoped that these points raised with regard to specific issues will encourage and stimulate practice developments in the fields of work concerned. However, we should supplement these specific aspects by considering more general suggestions concerning the translation of critical emancipatory theory into the reality of practice.

Again I must be very selective as there is so much that can be said about these issues, so many debates yet to be worked through. I shall therefore restrict myself to 14 particular comments, broken down into seven positive steps I feel need to be taken, and seven dangers to be avoided.

Positive steps

1   Much of the discrimination inherent in social work can be seen to be unintentional – due to a lack of awareness, rather than deliberate attempts to oppress. For this reason, awareness training has a major part to play (but this is not to be confused with the discredited Race Awareness Training – or RAT – discussed in Chapter 4). By bringing workers together in a training context, instances and issues of discrimi-nation can be identified and levels of awareness can thus be raised. Greater awareness at the **P** level can begin to undermine, to some limited degree at least, discriminatory culture and ideology at the **C** level. Awareness training therefore begins the process of challenging and confronting discrimination. It also acts as a foundation for other forms and levels of training.

2   The diversity approach is still in a relatively underdeveloped state, but we can none the less see the benefits of valuing diversity, of taking a broad-based, positive approach to tackling discrimination. The main advantage of the diversity approach is that it helps us to avoid the culture of defensiveness that has grown up around efforts to tackle discrimination and oppression (Thompson, 2009b).

3   Awareness training provides a consciousness-raising role for individu-als, but its value can be multiplied by raised collective awareness and subsequent collective action. Examples of alliances set up with this aim include: women's groups, race and culture groups, disability forums, equal opportunities monitoring groups. Recent years have seen a significant growth in the number and influence of such groups. A collective response to examples of discrimination can have a much more potent effect than an individual response. In addition, each individual can act with greater confidence in the knowledge that there exists the backing of others within a collective anti-discrimina-tory project.

4   Over 20 years ago Sibeon recognized the anti-intellectual tendencies in social work which devalue theory and advocate a 'common-sense'

approach to social work (Sibeon, 1991b), and the problems can be seen to continue to apply to this day (see Thompson, 2010). This is a particularly dangerous approach as far as anti-discriminatory practice is concerned. 'Common sense' amounts, in fact, to a mixture of dominant ideologies – and these often reflect sexist, racist and other discriminatory assumptions. It is a collection of taken-for-granted assumptions which have the potential to be discriminatory and oppressive in their content and impact (Thompson, 2000a). It is therefore essential that practice should be based on a clear and explicit theory base in order to be able to swim against the tide of dominant discriminatory assumptions. Anti-discriminatory social work therefore needs to be based on integrating theory and practice.

5   In order to develop emancipatory forms of practice we need to ensure that the issues and principles are seen as central – they are not an optional extra to be tagged on the end if time and resources permit. Equality, diversity and social justice should be central features of all social work theory, policy, education and practice. They need to be on the agenda for every service planning group, every working party, every course curriculum, every team philosophy and so on. Treating the subject as a separate, discrete area runs the risk of allowing it to become marginalized – a specialist subject for those who are interested, but not a mainstream issue. This is unacceptable, for, as we have seen, good practice must be anti-discriminatory practice.

6   Perhaps the most fundamental step towards anti-discriminatory practice that we can take is to become, and remain, open and critical in relation to our own practice (whether as direct practitioners, managers or educators). We need constantly to re-evaluate our practice and examine it in relation to our aims of challenging discrimination and thereby making a contribution to removing, reducing or alleviating oppression. The prefix 'anti' in anti-discriminatory practice is very significant; it denotes fighting against a powerful and established ideology. If we become complacent by failing to check that we are carrying through an emancipatory stance, discriminatory ideologies can subtly re-establish themselves in our thoughts and actions.

7   We can also promote anti-discriminatory practice by ensuring, as far as possible, that our actions are consistent with the principles of good practice more broadly. That is, if we wish to be well equipped to tackle discrimination and oppression, we need to ensure that we are not allowing other factors to undermine the quality and effectiveness of

our work. We therefore need to make sure that our practice is critically reflective, systematic and well-informed (see Thompson, 2015b, for a discussion of these issues).

Dangers

1 Anti-discriminatory practice challenges people's values and their taken-for-granted assumptions in constructing their own sense of reality. Such a challenge can prove very threatening and destabilizing. If not handled sensitively, exposure to anti-discriminatory ideas and values can prove so alien and threatening as to arouse considerable resistance and barriers to change. Too strong and insistent an approach is likely to be counterproductive and raise obstacles rather than awareness; indeed, it could be argued that an insensitive and overzealous approach to 'converting' others is not only a disservice to emancipatory practice but also a form of oppression in itself. If we are to avoid contributing to a culture of defensiveness, our focus needs to be on educating and convincing, not bullying.

2 The whole area of oppression and anti-discrimination is a complex and intricate field of study, with many contentious and problematic aspects. It is a political matter and therefore subject to competing values and interpretations. Consequently there can be no simple 'formula' solutions or easy answers. There are two interrelated dangers which arise from this: firstly, reductionism, the process of reducing a multifaceted, multilevel set of issues to a simple, single-level entity (for example, reducing **PCS** to personal prejudice); and, secondly, dogmatism, translating an open and dynamic theoretical system into a closed and static belief system or dogma.

3 Anti-discriminatory practice is indeed a complex area with many dimensions, such as race, gender, age and so on. One primary dimension which has received relatively little attention in this book is that of class. However, it has featured less here as it is more firmly established as a relevant factor in social work (due in no small part to the influence of the radical social work movement) and not because it is less important. A clear danger, therefore, is to fail to take account of the class dimension – the socioeconomic circumstances which: (a) underpin and magnify other forms of oppression; and (b) act as a major source of oppression in their own right. The danger, therefore, is one of going from a situation (for example, in the 1970s) where class was seen as

the primary, if not only, dimension of oppression to a situation in which it is barely considered (Jordan, 2000).

4 Class is part of the political underpinnings of anti-discriminatory practice and is also a key element in marxist theory which, in turn, is a central feature of radical social work. The influence of marxism has declined in recent years to be replaced, to a certain extent, by a neo-liberal philosophy which seeks to 'roll back the state' by lessening the state's role in welfare provision (Ferguson, 2008). The resulting privatization of welfare and its reliance on the profit motive are unlikely to provide fertile soil for the development of emancipatory forms of practice. Although the crude marxism of some aspects of 1960s and 1970s radicalism offered a far from adequate basis for social work, the rejection of a socialist political philosophy seriously weakens the scope for developing anti-discriminatory practice.

5 A further danger to be identified is that of 'colluding with the rhetoric'. What this means is that some people may use the right language and may make the right gestures, but without any underlying commitment to the values and principles of anti-discriminatory practice. They are just 'going through the motions', perhaps to avoid being branded as racist, sexist or whatever, or perhaps through confusion, ignorance or insecurity about how to practise in a genuinely anti-discriminatory way. This is a particularly worrying state of affairs, as it gives the impression that equality, diversity and social justice are being fostered when, in fact, inequalities are being maintained, condoned and reinforced.

6 A very significant danger is that of complacency. For example, I have encountered people who reject anti-discriminatory practice as being based on an exaggeration of the nature and extent of discrimination. We live in a mature democracy, they argue, and so discrimination cannot be as much of an issue as some people make out. This is a very naïve view which fails to take account of the extensive research base and the equally important base of the day-to-day experiences of social workers and clients. A variation on the complacency theme is the idea that, because we now have an extensive body of anti-discrimination legislation, the problems are of a fairly minor nature or extent. As we have seen, although the law can be very helpful, it has serious limitations when it comes to the complexities of discrimination and oppression.

7 Although not a widespread problem, the danger of competitiveness is still one worthy of mention. It is unfortunately the case that some

people see adopting a social justice perspective not so much as a foun dation of good practice or a moral-political imperative, but rather as a means to an end – to achieve promotion, obtain academic brownie points or whatever. While I have no objection to people having personal ambitions, it is sad that some people use an apparent commitment to justice and humanitarian values primarily for their own personal ends.

There are, of course, many other dangers and many other positive steps, some of which I have been able to pursue for further analysis in *Promoting Equality*. The points raised are intended not as a comprehensive overview, but rather as a set of pointers to guide and inform further discussion and action.

Social work is traditionally seen as operating on a knife edge of care and control. The discussions in this book, and more widely within the anti-discriminatory movement, not only recognize the significance of this knife edge but also relate it to another 'knife edge' situation. I am referring to the thin line between oppression and empowerment. That line also cuts through the centre of social work: the actions of social workers (and their agencies) are crucial in determining whether oppression is increased and strengthened or, alternatively, challenged and undermined through the process of empowerment.

Anti-discriminatory practice seeks to ensure that empowerment is to the fore in order to ensure that social work is a progressive force for social change and amelioration rather than a repressive arm of an uncaring state bureaucracy. The challenge is a major one, but the rewards for success are high, as indeed are the costs of failure.

REFERENCES

Abercrombie, N. and Warde, A., with Deem, R., Penna, S., Soothill, K., Urry, J., Sayer, A. and Walby, S. (2000) *Contemporary British Society*, 3rd edn, London, Polity.

Adams, R., Dominelli, L. and Payne, M. (eds) (2002) *Social Work: Themes, Issues and Critical Debates*, 2nd edn, Basingstoke, Palgrave Macmillan.

Ahmad, B. (1990) *Black Perspectives in Social Work*, Birmingham, Venture Press.

Alibhai-Brown, Y. (2001) *Mixed Feelings: The Complex Lives of Mixed-Race Britons*, London, The Women's Press.

Appignanesi, L. (2008) *Mad, Bad and Sad: A History of Women and the Mind Doctors from 1800 to the Present*, London, Virago.

Arber, S., Davidson, K. and Ginn, J. (eds) (2003) *Gender and Ageing: Changing Roles and Relationships*, Maidenhead, Open University Press.

Back, L. and Solomos, J. (eds) (2009) *Theories of Race and Racism: A Reader*, 2nd edn, London, Routledge.

Bailey, R. and Brake, N. (eds) (1975) *Radical Social Work*, London, Edward Arnold.

Baker, J., Lynch, K., Cantillon, S. and Walsh, J. (2004) *Equality: From Theory to Action*, Basingstoke, Palgrave Macmillan.

Banton, M. and Singh, G. (2014) '"Race", Disability and Oppression', in Swain et al. (2014).

Banyard, K. (2011) *The Equality Illusion: The Truth about Women and Men Today*, London, Faber & Faber.

Barker, C. (2008) *Cultural Studies*, 3rd edn, London, Sage.

Barnes, C. and Mercer, G. (2010) *Exploring Disability*, 2nd edn, Cambridge, Polity.

Barry, B. (2001) *Culture and Equality: An Egalitarian Critique of Multiculturalism*, Cambridge, Polity.

Barry, B. (2005) *Why Social Justice Matters*, Cambridge, Polity.

Bateman, N. (2008) 'Welfare Rights Practice', in Davies (2008).

Bauman, Z. (2000) *Modernity and the Holocaust*, 2nd edn, Cambridge, Polity.

Baxter, C. (ed.) (2001) *Managing Diversity and Inequality in Health Care*, London, Bailliere/Tindall.

Baxter, C., Poonia, K., Ward, L. and Nadirshaw, J. (1990) *Double Discrimination*, London, King's Fund Centre.

Beaumont, J. (2011) *Social Trends 41*, London, Office for National Statistics.

Beauvoir, S. de (1972) *The Second Sex*, Harmondsworth, Penguin.

Beauvoir, S. de (1977) *Old Age*, Harmondsworth, Penguin.

Bellin, W. (1994) 'Caring Professions and Welsh-speakers: A Perspective fror Language and Social Psychology', in Huws Williams, Williams and Davies (1994).

Bentall, R. P. (2004) *Madness Explained: Psychosis and Human Nature*, London, Penguin.

Bentall, R. P. (2010) *Doctoring the Mind: Why Psychiatric Treatments Fail*, London, Penguin.

Berger, P. L. (1966) *Invitation to Sociology*, Harmondsworth, Penguin.

Berger, P. L. and Luckmann, T. (1967) *The Social Construction of Reality*, Harmondsworth, Penguin.

Bernard, M. and Scharf, T. (eds) (2009) *Critical Perspectives on Ageing Societies*, Bristol, The Policy Press.

Bevan, D. (1998) 'Death, Dying and Inequality', *Care: The Journal of Practice and Development* 7(1).

Bevan, D. (2002) 'Poverty and Deprivation', in Thompson (2002b).

Bhat A., Carr-Hill, R. and Ohri, S. (eds) (1988) *Britain's Black Population: A New Perspective*, Aldershot, Gower.

Bhatti-Sinclair, K. (2011) *Anti-Racist Practice in Social Work*, Basingstoke, Palgrave Macmillan.

Blackburn, D. G. (2000) 'Why Race Is Not a Biological Concept', in Lang (2000).

Board for Social Responsibility (1990) *Ageing*, London, Church House Publishing.

Bolton, S. C. (ed.) (2007) *Dimensions of Dignity at Work*, London, Butterworth-Heinemann.

Bond, J. and Cabrero, G. R. (2007) 'Health and Dependency in Later Life', in Bond et al. (2007).

Bond, J. and Coleman, P. (eds) (1990) *Ageing in Society – An Introduction to Social Gerontology*, London, Sage.

Bond, J., Peace, S., Dittmann-Kohli, F. and Westerhof, G. (eds) (2007) *Ageing in Society: European Perspectives on Gerontology*, 3rd edn, London, Sage.

Bottomore, T. B. and Rubel, M. (eds) (1963) *Selected Writings in Sociology and Social Philosophy*, Harmondsworth, Penguin.

Boyle, M. (2002) *Schizophrenia: A Scientific Delusion?*, 2nd edn, London, Routledge.

Brearley, C. P. (1982) *Risk and Ageing*, London, Routledge & Kegan Paul.

Brewer, J. D. (1991) 'The Parallels Between Sectarianism and Racism: The Northern Ireland Experience', in CD Project Steering Group (1991).

Brisenden, S. (1986) 'Independent Living and the Medical Model of Disability', *Disability, Handicap and Society* 1(2).

Brown, H. C. and Cocker, C. (2011) *Social Work with Lesbians and Gay Men*, London, Sage.

Brown, G. W. and Harris, T. (1978) *The Social Origins of Depression*, London, Tavistock.

Bryson, V. (1999) *Feminist Debates: Issues of Theory and Political Practice*, Basingstoke, Macmillan Press [now Palgrave Macmillan].

REFERENCES

llock, A. and Trombley, S. (eds) (2000) *The New Fontana Dictionary of Modern Thought*, 3rd edn, London, HarperCollins.

ulmer, M. (2010) 'Measuring Race and Ethnicity', in Bulmer, Gibbs and Hyman (2010).

Bulmer, M., Gibbs, J. and Hyman, L. (eds) (2010) *Social Measurement through Social Surveys: An Applied Approach*, Farnham, Ashgate.

Burke, B. and Harrison, P. (2000) 'Race and Racism in Social Work', in Davies (2000).

Burr, V. (2003) *Social Constructionism*, 2nd edn, London, Routledge.

Busfield, J. (1986) *Managing Madness: Changing Ideas and Practice*, London, Hutchinson.

Butler, J. (2006) *Gender Trouble*, London, Routledge.

Butler, R. N. (1975) *Why Survive? Being Old in America*, New York, Harper & Row.

Bytheway, W. R. and Johnson, J. (1990) 'On Defining Ageism', *Critical Social Policy 29*.

Cameron, C. (2014) *Disability Studies: A Student's Guide*, London, Sage.

Canavan, S. and Prior, S. (2008) 'Sexuality and Sexual Relationships', in Davies (2008).

Cann, P. and Dean, M. (eds) (2009) *Unequal Ageing: The Untold Story of Exclusion in Old Age*, Bristol, the Policy Press.

Carabine, J. (2004a) 'Sexualities, Personal Lives and Social Policy', in Carabine (2004b).

Carabine, J. (ed.) (2004b) *Sexualities: Personal Lives and Social Policy*, Bristol, The Policy Press.

Care Council for Wales (2010) *They All Speak English Anyway*, Cardiff, Care Council for Wales.

Carlen, P. and Worrall, A. (eds) (1987) *Gender, Crime and Justice*, Milton Keynes, Open University Press.

Carter, H. and Aitchison, J. (1986) 'Language Areas and Language Change in Wales: 1961–1991', in Hume and Pryce (1986).

Cattan, M. (2009) *Mental Health and Well-Being in Later Life*, Maidenhead, Open University Press.

CD Project Steering Group (eds) (1991) *Setting the Context for Change*, London, CCETSW.

Chadwick, A. (1996) 'Knowledge, Power and the Disability Discrimination Bill', *Disability and Society* 11(1).

Chakrabarti, M. (1990) 'Racial Prejudice' Open University, Workbook 6, Part 1 of K254, *Working with Children and Young People*.

Chamberlin, J. (2006) 'Foreword', in Thornicroft (2006).

Christie, A. (ed.) (2001) *Men and Social Work: Theories and Practices*, Basingstoke, Palgrave Macmillan.

Clarke, V., Ellis, S. J., Peel, E. and Riggs, D. W. (2010) *Lesbian, Gay, Bisexual, Trans and Queer Psychology: An Introduction*, Cambridge, Cambridge University Press.

Clarke, J. and Cochrane, A. (1998) 'The Social Construction of Social Problems', Saraga (1998).

Clements, L. and Read, J. (2003) *Disabled People and European Human Rights*, Bristol, The Policy Press.

Cocker, C. and Hafford-Letchfield, T. (2010) 'Critical Commentary: Out and Proud? Social Work's Relationship with Lesbian and Gay Equality', *British Journal of Social Work* 40(6).

Cohen, C. I. and Timini, S. (eds) (2008) *Liberatory Psychiatry: Philosophy, Politics and Mental Health*, Cambridge, Cambridge University Press.

Cohen, M. B. and Mullender, A. (eds) (2002) *Gender and Groupwork*, London, Routledge.

Cohen, P. N. and MacCartney, D. (2007) 'Inequality and the Family', in Scott, Treas and Richards (2007).

Cole, M. (ed.) (2011) *Education, Equality and Human Rights: Issues of Gender, 'Race', Sexual Orientation, Disability and Social Class*, London, Routledge.

Collins, P. H. (2000) *Black Feminist Thought: Knowledge, Consciousness, and the Politics of Empowerment*, London, Routledge.

Collins, P. H. (2011) 'Black Feminist Epistemology and Towards a Politics of Empowerment', in Cree (2011).

The Commission on British Muslims and Islamophobia (ed.) (2004) *Islamophobia: Issues, Challenges and Action*, Stoke-on-Trent, Trentham Books.

Coombe, V. and Little, A. (eds) (1986) *Race and Social Work: A Guide to Training*, London, Tavistock Publications.

Corby, B. (1989) 'Alternative Theory Bases in Child Abuse', in Stainton Rogers et al. (1989).

Coulshed, V. and Mullender, A. with Jones, D. and Thompson, N. (2006) *Management in Social Work*, 3rd edn, Basingstoke, Palgrave Macmillan.

Cree, V. (ed.) (2011) *Social Work: A Reader*, London, Routledge.

Crossley, N. (2006) *Contesting Psychiatry: Social Movements in Mental Health*, London, Routledge.

Dallos, R. and McLaughlin, E. (eds) (1993) *Social Problems and the Family*, London, Sage.

Dalrymple, J. and Burke, B. (2006) *Anti-Oppressive Practice, Social Care and the Law*, 2nd edn, Maidenhead, Open University Press.

Davies, E. (2009) *Different Words, Different Worlds: The Concept of Language Choice in Social Work and Social Care*, Cardiff, Care Council for Wales.

Davies, M. (ed.) (2000) *The Blackwell Encyclopaedia of Social Work*, Oxford, Blackwell.

Davies, M. (ed.) (2008) *The Blackwell Companion to Social Work*, 3rd edn, Oxford, Blackwell.

Davies, S. G. (2007) *Challenging Gender Norms: Five Genders Among Bugis in Indonesia*, Belmont, CA, Thomson Wadsworth.

Davis, K. (1988) 'Issues in Disability: Integrated Living', Open University, Unit 19 of D211 *Social Problems and Social Welfare*.

REFERENCES

is, K. (1996) 'Disability and Legislation: Rights and Equality', in Hales (1996).

DP (1985) 'Development of the Derbyshire Centre for Integrated Living', Chesterfield, Derbyshire Coalition of Disabled People.

DePalma, R. and Atkinson, E. (eds) (2008) *Invisible Boundaries: Addressing Sexualities Equality in Children's Worlds*, Stoke-on-Trent, Trentham Books.

Divine, D. (1990) 'Sharing the Struggle', *Social Work Today*, 22 November.

Dobelniece, S. (1998) 'Poverty and Deprivation', in Lešnik (1998).

Doka, K. J. and Martin, T. L. (2010) *Grieving Beyond Gender: Understanding the Ways Women Mourn*, London, Routledge.

Dominelli, L. (2002) *Anti-Oppressive Social Work Theory and Practice*, Basingstoke, Palgrave Macmillan.

Dorling, D. (2014) *Inequality and the 1%*, London, Verso.

Dorling, D. (2015) *Injustice: Why Social Inequality Still Persists*, 2nd edn, Bristol, The Policy Press.

Drakeford, M. and Morris, S. (1998) 'Social Work with Linguistic Minorities', in Williams, Soydan and Johnson (1998).

Edmondoson, R. and Kondratowitz, H.-J. von (eds) (2009) *Valuing Older People: A Humanist Approach to Ageing*, Bristol, The Policy Press.

Ellison, G. and Gunstone, B. (2009) *Sexual Orientation Explored: A Study of Identity, Attraction, Behaviour and Attitudes in 2009*, Manchester, Equality and Human Rights Commission.

Engels, F. (1976) *The Origin of the Family, Private Property and the State*, London, Lawrence & Wishart [originally published 1844].

Equality and Human Rights Commission (2009) *Beyond Tolerance: Making Sexual Orientation a Public Matter*, Manchester, Equality and Human Rights Commission.

Farrell, F. and Watt, P. (eds) (2001) *Responding to Racism in Ireland*, Dublin, Veritas.

Fawcett, B. and Karban, K. (2005) *Contemporary Mental Health: Theory, Policy and Practice*, London, Routledge.

Featherstone, M. and Hepworth, M. (1990) 'Images of Ageing', in Bond and Coleman (1990).

Fennell, G., Phillipson, C. and Evers, H. (1988) *The Sociology of Old Age*, Milton Keynes, Open University Press.

Ferguson, I. (2008) *Reclaiming Social Work: Challenging Neo-liberalism and Promoting Social Justice*, London, Sage.

Ferguson, I. and Woodward, R. (2009) *Radical Social Work in Practice: Making a Difference*, Bristol, The Policy Press.

Fernando, S. (2010) *Mental Health, Race and Culture*, 3rd edn, Basingstoke, Palgrave Macmillan.

Finch, J. and Groves, D. (eds) (1983) *A Labour of Love*, London, Routledge & Kegan Paul.

Fine, C. (2011) *Delusions of Gender: The Real Science Behind Sex Differences*, London, Icon Books.

Finkelstein, V. (1981) 'Disability and Professional Attitudes', Sevenoaks, NAIDEX Convention.

REFERENCES

Finkelstein, V. (2004) 'Representing Disability', in Swain et al. (2014).

Fischer, A. (ed.) (2000) *Gender and Emotion: Social Psychological Perspectiv* Cambridge, Cambridge University Press.

Fisher, M. (1994) 'Man-made Care: Community Care and Older Male Carers', *British Journal of Social Work* 24(6): 659–80.

Foucault, M. (1977) *Discipline and Punish: The Birth of the Prison*, London, Allen Lane.

Foucault, M. (1979) *The History of Sexuality. Volume 1: An Introduction*, London, Allen Lane.

Frazer, H. (2001) 'Racism, Poverty and Community Development', in Farrell and Watt (2001).

Freire, P. (1972) *Pedagogy of the Oppressed*, Harmondsworth, Penguin.

Fröschl, E. (2002) 'The Social Work Profession', in Gruber and Stefanov (2002).

Furness, S. and Gilligan, P. (2009) *Religion, Belief and Social Work*, Bristol, The Policy Press.

Gambrill, E. (2005) 'Critical Thinking, Evidence-Based Practice, and Mental Health', in Kirk (2005).

Garrett, P. M. (2002) 'Social Work and the Just Society: Diversity, Difference and the Sequestration of Poverty', *Journal of Social Work* 2(2).

Garrett, P. M. (2004) *Social Work and Irish People in Britain: Historical and Contemporary Responses to Irish Children and Families*, Bristol, The Policy Press.

Gauntlett, D. (2002) *Media, Gender and Identity: An Introduction*, London, Routledge.

Giddens, A. (1971) *Capitalism and Modern Social Theory*, Cambridge, Cambridge University Press.

Giddens, A. (2009) *Sociology*, 6th edn, Cambridge, Polity.

Gilleard, C. and Higgs, P. (2005) *Contexts of Ageing: Class, Cohort and Community*, Cambridge, Polity.

Gilleat-Ray, S. (2010) *Muslims in Britain: An Introduction*, Cambridge, Cambridge University Press.

Goodley, D. (2011) *Disability Studies: An Interdisciplinary Introduction*, London, Sage.

Gott, M. and Hinchliff, S. (2003) 'Sex and Ageing: A Gendered Issue', in Arber, Davidson and Ginn (2003).

Graham, M. (2002) *Social Work and African-Centred Worldviews*, Birmingham, Venture Press.

Green, T. H. (2015) *Fear of Islam: An Introduction to Islamophobia in the West*, Minneapolis, MN, Fortress Press.

Gruber, C. and Stefanov, H. (eds) (2002) *Gender in Social Work: Promoting Equality*, Lyme Regis, Russell House Publishing.

Hales, G. (ed.) (1996) *Beyond Disability: Towards an Enabling Society*, London, Sage.

Halmos, P. (1965) *The Faith of the Counsellors*, London, Constable.

Hans, A. and A. Patri (eds) (2003) *Women, Disability and Identity*, New Delhi, Sage.

REFERENCES

ne, O. and Dickson, D. (eds) (2003) *Researching the Troubles*, Edinburgh, Mainstream Publishing.

ne, L. and Radford, J. (2008) *Tackling Domestic Violence: Theories, Policies and Practice*, Maidenhead, Open University Press.

Iarris, V. (1991) 'Values of Social Work in the Context of British Society in Conflict with Anti-Racism', in CD Project Steering Group (1991).

Hayward, S. (2005) *Women Leading*, Basingstoke, Palgrave Macmillan.

Hechter, M. (1999) *Internal Colonialism: The Celtic Fringe in British National Development 1536–1966*, 2nd edn, London, Routledge.

Heenan, D. and Birrell, D. (2011) *Social Work in Northern Ireland: Conflict and Change*, Bristol, The Policy Press.

Heidegger, M. (1962) *Being and Time*, Oxford, Blackwell [originally published 1927].

Hill Collins, P. (2009) 'Black Feminist Thought', in Back and Solomos (2009).

Hills, J. (2015) *Good Times, Bad Times: The Welfare Myth of Them and Us*, Bristol, The Policy Press.

Hockey, J. and James, A. (1993) *Growing Up and Growing Old: Ageing and Dependency in the Life Course*, London, Sage.

Hocquenghem, G. (1978) *Homosexual Desire*, London, Allison & Busby.

Hodges, I. (2008) 'Queer Dilemmas: The Problem of Power in Psychotherapeutic and Counselling Practice', in Moon (2008).

Holloway, M. and Moss, B. (2010) *Spirituality and Social Work*, Basingstoke, Palgrave Macmillan.

Hooks, B. (1982) *Ain't I a Woman: Black Women and Feminism*, London, Pluto.

Hooks, B. (1986) 'Sisterhood: Political Solidarity Between Women', *Feminist Review* 23.

Hornstein, Z. (ed.) (2001) *Outlawing Age Discrimination: Foreign Lessons, UK Choices*, Bristol, The Policy Press.

Hughes, B. and Mtezuka, E. M. (1992) 'Social Work and Older Women', in Langan and Day (1992).

Hughes, G. (1998) 'A Suitable Case for Treatment', in Saraga (1998).

Hugman, R. (1994) *Ageing and the Care of Older People in Europe*, Basingstoke, Macmillan Press [now Palgrave Macmillan].

Hume, I. and Pryce, W. T. R. (eds) (1986) *The Welsh and Their Country*, Llandysul, Dyfed, Gomer.

Hunt, R. and Jensen, J. (2007) *The School Report: The Experiences of Young Gay People in Britain's Schools*, London, Stonewall [www.stonewall.org.uk/education_for_all/research/1790.asp].

Husband, C. (1986) 'Racism, Prejudice and Social Policy', in Coombe and Little (1986).

Hussain, D. (2008) 'Islam', in Lodge and Cooper (2008).

Huws Williams, R., Williams, H. and Davies, E. (eds) (1994) *Gwaith Cymdeithasol a'r Iaith Gymraeg/Social Work and the Welsh Language*, Cardiff, University of Wales Press.

REFERENCES

Ives, K. (2007) *Cixous, Irigaray, Kristeva: The Jouissance of French Feminism*, edn, Maidstone, Crescent Moon.

Jack, R. (1995a) 'Introduction', in Jack (1995b).

Jack, R. (ed.) (1995b) *Empowerment in Community Care*, London, Chapman & Hall.

Jansz, J. (2000) 'Masculine Identity and Restrictive Emotionality', in Fischer (2000).

Jivraj, S. and Simpson, L. (eds) (2015) *Ethnic Identity and Inequalities in Britain*, Bristol, The Policy Press.

Jones, O. (2015) *The Establishment and How They Get Away with It*, London, Penguin.

Jordan, B. (2000) *Social Work and the Third Way*, London, Sage.

Joseph, J. E. (2004) *Language and Identity: National, Ethnic, Religious*, Basingstoke, Palgrave Macmillan.

Kaltner, J. (2003) *Islam: What Non-Muslims Should Know*, Minneapolis, MN, Fortress.

Kandola, R. and Fullerton, J. (1998) *Diversity in Action: Managing the Mosaic*, 2nd edn, London, Chartered Institute of Personnel and Development.

Katz, J. (1978) *White Awareness*, Norman, University of Oklahoma Press.

Kirk, S. A. (ed.) (2005) *Mental Disorders in the Social Environment: Critical Perspectives*, New York, Columbia University Press.

Kirk, S. A., Gomory, T. and Cohen, D. (2015) *Mad Science: Psychiatric Coercion, Diagnosis and Drugs*, Piscataway, NJ, Transaction Publishers.

Kirton, D. (2000) *'Race', Ethnicity and Adoption*, Buckingham, Open University Press.

Kundnani, A. (2015) *The Muslims Are Coming!: Islamophobia, Extremism and the Domestic War on Terror*, London, Verso.

Laing, R. D. (1965) *The Divided Self*, Harmondsworth, Penguin.

Laing, R. D. (1967) *The Politics of Experience and the Bird of Paradise*, Harmondsworth, Penguin.

Laing, R. D. and Cooper, D. (1971) *Reason and Violence*, London, Tavistock.

Laird, S. E. (2008) *Anti-Oppressive Social Work: A Guide for Developing Cultural Competence*, London, Sage.

Lance, M. N. (2005) 'Identity Judgements, Queer Politics', in Morland and Willox (2005).

Lang, B. (ed.) (2000) *Race and Racism in Theory and Practice*, Lanham, MD, Rowman & Littlefield.

Langan, M. and Day, L. (eds) (1992) *Women, Oppression and Social Work: Issues in Anti-discriminatory Practice*, London, Routledge.

Lansley, S. and Mack, J. (2015) *Breadline Britain: The Rise of Mass Poverty*, London, Oneworld Publications.

Lawler, S. (2008) *Identity: Sociological Perspectives*, Cambridge, Polity.

Leonard, P. (1975) 'Towards a Paradigm for Radical Practice', in Bailey and Brake (1975).

Lešnik, B. (ed.) (1998) *Countering Discrimination in Social Work*, Aldershot, Arena.

Lin, N. (2002) *Social Capital: A Theory of Social Structure and Action*, Cambridge, Cambridge University Press.

, R. (2003) *Citizenship: Feminist Perspectives*, 2nd edn, Basingstoke, Palgrave Macmillan.

er, R. (2004) *Poverty*, 2nd edn, Cambridge, Polity.

yd, M. (2001) 'The Politics of Disability and Feminism: Discord or Synthesis', *Sociology* 35(3).

Lodge, G. and Cooper, Z. (eds) (2008) *Faith in the Nation: Religion, Identity and the Public Realm in Britain*, London, IPPR.

Lonsdale, S. (1990) *Women and Disability*, Basingstoke, Macmillan Press [now Palgrave Macmillan].

Luck, M., Bamford, M. and Williamson, P. (2000) *Men's Health: Perspectives, Diversity and Paradox*, Oxford, Blackwell.

Macpherson, W. (1999) *The Stephen Lawrence Inquiry: Report of an Inquest*, London, Stationery Office.

Malik, K, (2008) *Strange Fruit: Why Both Sides Are Wrong in the Race Debate*, Oxford, Oneworld Publications.

Mandelbaum, D. G. (ed.) (1949) *Selected Writings of Edward Sapir: A Study in Phonetic Symbolism*, Berkeley, CA, University of California.

Marks, D. (2000) 'Disability', in Davies (2000).

Marlow, A. and Loveday, B. (eds) (2000) *After Macpherson: Policing After the Stephen Lawrence Inquiry*, Lyme Regis, Russell House Publishing.

Marshall, V. W. (1986a) 'A Sociological Perspective on Aging and Dying', in Marshall (1986b).

Marshall, V. W. (1986b) *Later Life: The Social Psychology of Aging*, London, Sage.

May, M., Page, R. and Brunsdon, E. (eds) (2001) *Understanding Social Problems: Issues in Social Policy*, Oxford, Blackwell.

Mende, A. von and Houlihan, M. (2007) 'The Dignity of Difference? Experiences of Foreign Workers in the Multicultural Workplace', in Bolton (2007).

Mercer, G. (2014) 'User-Led Organizations: Facilitating Independent Living', in Swain et al. (2014).

Midwinter, E. (1990) 'An Ageing World: The Equivocal Response', *Ageing and Society* 10.

Millar, R. M. (2005) *Language, Nation and Power: An Introduction*, Basingstoke, Palgrave Macmillan.

Millett, K. (1971) *Sexual Politics*, London, Rupert Hart-Davis.

Mills, C. W. (1970) *The Sociological Imagination*, Harmondsworth, Penguin.

Milner, J. and O'Byrne, P. (2009) *Assessment in Social Work*, 3rd edn, Basingstoke, Palgrave Macmillan.

Moon, L. (ed.) (2008) *Feeling Queer or Queer Feelings? Radical Approaches to Counselling, Sex, Sexualities and Genders*, London, Routledge.

Mooney, A. and Evans, B. (2015) *Language, Society and Power: An Introduction*, 4th edn, London, Routledge.

Morgan, C., Dazzan, P., Morgan, K., Jones, P., Harrison, G., Leff, J. Murray, R. and Fearon, P. (2006) 'First Episode Psychoses and Ethnicity: Initial Findings from the AESOP Study', *World Psychiatry* 5(1).

Morgan, K. O. (1982) *Rebirth of a Nation: Wales 1880–1980*, Oxford Univer Press/University of Wales Press.

Morland, I. and Willox, A. (eds) (2005) *Queer Theory*, Basingstoke, Palgrav Macmillan.

Morris, J. (1991) *Pride Against Prejudice*, London, Women's Press.

Moss, B. (2005) *Religion and Spirituality*, Lyme Regis, Russell House Publishing.

Moss, B. (2007) *Values*, Lyme Regis, Russell House Publishing.

Moss, B. and Thompson, N. (2007) 'Spirituality and Equality', *Social & Public Policy Review* 1(1).

Muldoon, J. (2000) 'Race or Culture: Medieval Notions of Difference', in Lang (2000).

Mullaly, B. (2009) *Challenging Oppression and Countering Privilege*, 2nd edn Oxford, Oxford University Press.

Mullender, A. (2008) 'Engendering The Social Work Agenda', in Davies (2008).

Munro, A. and McCulloch, W. (1969) *Psychiatry for Social Workers*, Oxford, Pergamon Press.

Neal, S., Bennett, K., Cochrane, A. and Mahon, G. (2013) 'Living Multiculture: Understanding the New Spatial and Social Relations of Ethnicity and Multiculture in England', *Environment and Planning C: Government and Policy,* 31(2).

Netmetz, P. L. and Christensen, S. L. (1996) 'The Challenge of Cultural Diversity: Harnessing a Diversity of Views to Understand Multiculturalism', *Academy of Management Review* 21(2).

Nolan, M., Davies, S. and Grant, G. (eds) (2001) *Working with Older People: Key Issues in Policy and Practice*, Buckingham, Open University Press.

Norman, A. (1980) *Rights and Risk*, London, Centre for Policy on Ageing.

Norman, A. (1987) 'Overcoming an Old Prejudice', *Community Care*, 29 January.

Oliver, M. (1990) *The Politics of Disablement*, Basingstoke, Macmillan [now Palgrave Macmillan].

Oliver, M. (2009) *Understanding Disability: From Theory to Practice*, 2nd edn, Basingstoke, Palgrave Macmillan.

Oliver, M. and Barnes, C. (2012) *The Politics of Disablement*, 2nd edn, London, Palgrave Macmillan.

Oliver, M., Sapey, B. and Thomas, P. (2012) *Social Work with Disabled People*, 4th edn, Basingstoke, Palgrave Macmillan.

Ong, B. N. (1985) 'The Paradox of "Wonderful Children": The Case of Child Abuse', *Early Childhood Development and Care* 21.

Owen, C. and Statham, J. (2009) *Disproportionality in Child Welfare: The Prevalence of Black and Minority Ethnic Children within the 'Looked After' and 'Children in Need' Populations and on Child Protection Registers in England*, London: Department for Children, Schools and Families.

Parekh, B. (2006) *Rethinking Multiculturalism: Cultural Diversity and Political Thinking*, 2nd edn, Basingstoke, Palgrave Macmillan.

Parekh, B. (2008) *A New Politics of Identity: Political Principles for an Interdependent World*, Basingstoke, Palgrave Macmillan.

REFERENCES

, J. W. (2011) *The End of Sexual Identity: Why Sex is Too Important to Define What We Are*, Downers Grove, IL, IVP Books.

ton, C. and Parton, N. (1989) 'Women, the Family and Child Protection', *Critical Social Policy* 24.

arton, N. and O'Byrne, P. (2000) *Constructive Social Work: Towards a New Practice*, Basingstoke, Macmillan Press [now Palgrave Macmillan].

Pascall, G. (1997) *Social Policy: A New Feminist Analysis*, London, Routledge.

Payne, G. (2006) *Social Divisions*, 2nd edn, Basingstoke, Palgrave Macmillan.

Pearson, G. (1975) *The Deviant Imagination*, Basingstoke, Macmillan Press [now Palgrave Macmillan].

Penketh, L. (2000) *Tackling Institutional Racism*, Bristol, The Policy Press.

Phillipson, C. (1982) *Capitalism and the Construction of Old Age*, Basingstoke, Macmillan Press [now Palgrave Macmillan].

Phillipson, C. (2000) 'Ageism', in Davies (2000).

Pickering, M. (2001) *Stereotyping: The Politics of Representation*, Basingstoke, Palgrave Macmillan.

Pilcher, J. and Whelehan, I. (2004) *50 Key Concepts in Gender Studies*, London, Sage.

Pilkington, A. (2003) *Racial Disadvantage and Ethnic Diversity in Britain*, Basingstoke, Palgrave Macmillan.

Pincus, F. L. (2011) *Understanding Diversity: An Introduction to Class, Race, Gender, and Sexual Orientation*, 2nd edn, Boulder, CO, Lynne Rienner.

Powell, J. L. (2006) *Social Theory and Aging*, New York, Rowman & Littlefield.

Powell, J. L. and Chamberlain, J. M. (2012) *Social Welfare, Aging and Social Theory*, Lanham, MD, Lexington Books.

Prevatt Goldstein, B. (2008) 'Black Perspectives', in Davies (2008).

Pullen, A., Beech, N. and Sims, D. (eds) (2007) *Exploring Identity: Concepts and Methods*, Basingstoke, Palgrave Macmillan.

Radford, L. (2001) 'Domestic Violence', in May, Page and Brunsdon (2001).

Ramazanoglu, C. (1989) *Feminism and the Contradictions of Oppression*, London, Routledge.

Richardson, D. and Robinson, V. (eds) (2007) *Introducing Gender and Women's Studies*, 3rd edn, Basingstoke, Palgrave Macmillan.

Riches, G. (2002) 'Gender', in Thompson (2002b).

Ridge, T. and Wright, S. (eds) (2008) *Understanding Inequality, Poverty and Wealth: Policies and Prospects*, Bristol, The Policy Press.

Roberts, K. (2011) *Class in Contemporary Britain*, 2nd edn, Basingstoke, Palgrave Macmillan.

Robertson, S. (2014) 'Men and Disability', in Swain et al. (2014).

Robinson, L. (2002) 'Social Work through the Life Course', in Adams, Dominelli, and Payne (2002).

Robinson, L. (2008) *Psychology for Social Workers: Black Perspectives*, 2nd edn, London, Routledge.

Rojek, C., Peacock, G. and Collins, S. (1988) *Social Work and Received Ideas*, London, Routledge.

REFERENCES

Rooney, B. (1987) *Racism and Resistance to Change*, Liverpool, Merseyside
Profile Group.

Rowbotham, S. (1973) *Woman's Consciousness, Man's World*, Harmondsworth,
Penguin.

Roys, P. (1988) 'Social Services', in Bhat, Carr-Hill and Ohri (1988).

Runnymede Trust (1997) *Islamophobia: A Challenge for Us All* [www.runnymede
trust.org].

Rush, F. (1981) *The Best Kept Secret*, Englewood Cliffs, NJ, Prentice-Hall.

Ryan, W. (1988) *Blaming the Victim*, 2nd edn, New York, Random House.

Saleebey, D. (2006) *The Strengths Perspective in Social Work Practice*, 4th edn,
Boston, MA, Pearson Education.

Sanders, S. (2008) 'Tackling Homophobia, Creating Safer Spaces', in DePalma and
Atkinson (2008).

Sapey, B. (2002) 'Disability', in Thompson (2002b).

Sapey, B. (2004) 'Impairment, Disability and Loss: Reassessing the Rejection of
Loss', *Illness, Crisis & Loss* 12(1).

Saraga, E. (1993) 'The Abuse of Children', in Dallos and McLaughlin (1993).

Saraga, E. (ed.) (1998) *Embodying the Social: Constructions of Difference*, London,
Routledge.

Sargeant, M. (ed.) (2011) *Age Discrimination and Diversity: Multiple Discrimination
from An Age Perspective*, Cambridge, Cambridge University Press.

Sartre, J-P. (1976) *Critique of Dialectical Reason*, London, Verso.

Scharf, T. (2009) 'Too Tight to Mention: Unequal Income in Older Age', in Cann
and Dean (2009).

SCIE (2006) *Dignity in Care: Adults' Services Practice Guide*, London, Social Care
Institute for Excellence.

Scott, J., Treas, J. and Richards, M. (eds) (2007) *The Blackwell Companion to the
Sociology of Families*, Oxford, Blackwell.

Segal, L. (1999) *Why Feminism?*, Cambridge, Polity.

Segal, L. (2007) *Slow Motion: Changing Masculinities, Changing Men*, 3rd edn,
Basingstoke, Palgrave Macmillan.

Shah, N. A. (2006) 'Women's Rights in the Koran: An Interpretive Approach',
Human Rights Quarterly 28(4).

Shakespeare, T. (2013) *Disability Rights and Wrongs Revisited*, 2nd edn, London,
Routledge.

Sheldon, A. (1999) 'Personal and Perplexing: Feminist Disability Politics Evaluated',
Disability and Society 14(5).

Sheldon, A. (2014) 'Women and Disability', in Swain et al. (2014).

Sibeon, R. (1991a) 'Emancipatory theories, policies and practices in a welfare
profession: an anti-reductionist perspective on social work politics', paper
presented at the British Sociological Association Annual Conference,
Manchester.

Sibeon, R. (1991b) *Towards a New Sociology of Social Work*, Aldershot, Avebury.

Sibeon, R. (2004) *Rethinking Social Theory*, London, Sage.

REFERENCES

, M. (1995) *Health in Old Age: Myth, Mystery and Management*, Buckingham, Open University Press.

erman, P. and Berzoff, J. (eds) (2004) *Living with Dying*, New York, Columbia University Press.

mpson, P. (2015) *Middle-Aged Men, Ageing and Ageism: Over the Rainbow?*, London, Palgrave Macmillan.

Sivanandan, A. (1991) 'Black Struggles Against Racism', in CD Project Steering Group (1991).

Smart, N. (1998) *The World's Religions*, Cambridge, Cambridge University Press.

Solomos, J. (2003) *Race and Racism in Contemporary Britain*, 3rd edn, Basingstoke, Palgrave Macmillan.

Sone, A. (1991) 'Outward Bound', *Community Care*, 8 August.

Soydan, H. and Williams, C. (1998) 'Exploring Concepts', in Williams, Soydan, and Johnson (1998).

Spicker, P. (2001) 'Income and Wealth', in May, Page and Brunsdon (2001).

Stepney, P. and Ford, D. (eds) (2011) *Social Work Models, Methods and Theories: A Framework for Practice*, 2nd edn, Lyme Regis, Russell House Publishing.

Stiglitz, J. E. (2013) *The Price of Inequality*, London, Penguin.

Swain, J., French, S., Barnes, C. and Thomas, C. (eds) (2014) *Disabling Barriers – Enabling Environments*, 3rd edn, London, Sage.

Tanner, D. (2010) *Managing the Ageing Experience: Learning from Older People*, Bristol, The Policy Press.

Tew, J. (2011) *Social Approaches to Mental Distress*, Basingstoke, Palgrave Macmillan.

Thompson, N. (1992) *Existentialism and Social Work*, Aldershot, Avebury.

Thompson, N. (1995a) *Age and Dignity: Working with Older People*, Aldershot, Arena.

Thompson, N. (1995b) 'Men and Anti-Sexism', *British Journal of Social Work* 25(4).

Thompson, N. (1998) 'Towards a Theory of Emancipatory Practice', in Lešnik (1998).

Thompson, N. (2000a) *Theory and Practice in Human Services*, 2nd edn, Buckingham, Open University Press.

Thompson, N. (2000b) *Tackling Bullying and Harassment in the Workplace*, Birmingham, Pepar.

Thompson, N. (2002a) *Building the Future: Social Work with Children, Young People and Their Families*, Lyme Regis, Russell House Publishing.

Thompson, N. (ed.) (2002b) *Loss and Grief: A Guide for Human Services Practitioners*, Basingstoke, Palgrave Macmillan.

Thompson, N. (2002c) 'Social Work with Adults', in Adams, Dominelli and Payne (2002).

Thompson, N. (2007) *Power and Empowerment*, Lyme Regis, Russell House Publishing.

Thompson, N. (2008) 'Anti-Discriminatory Practice', in Davies (2008).

REFERENCES

Thompson, N. (2009a) *Practising Social Work: Meeting the Professional Cha* Basingstoke, Palgrave Macmillan.

Thompson, N. (2009b) *Promoting Equality, Valuing Diversity: A Learning Development Manual*, Lyme Regis, Russell House Publishing.

Thompson, N. (2010) *Theorizing Social Work Practice*, Basingstoke, Palgrave Macmillan.

Thompson, N. (2011a) *Promoting Equality: Working with Diversity and Difference*, 3rd edn, Basingstoke, Palgrave Macmillan.

Thompson, N. (2011b) *Effective Communication: A Guide for the People Professions*, 2nd edn, Basingstoke, Palgrave Macmillan.

Thompson, N. (2011c) *Crisis Intervention*, Lyme Regis, Russell House Publishing.

Thompson, N. (2012) 'Existentialist Practice', in Stepney and Ford (2012).

Thompson, N. (2015a) *People Skills*, 4th edn, London, Palgrave Macmillan.

Thompson, N. (2015b) *Understanding Social Work: Preparing for Practice*, 4th edn, London, Palgrave Macmillan.

Thompson, N. and Bates, J. (2002) 'Men, Masculinity and Social Work', in Gruber and Stefanov (2002).

Thompson, N. and Thompson, S. (2001) 'Empowering Older People: Beyond the Care Model', *Journal of Social Work* 1(1).

Thompson, N. and Thompson, S. (2004) 'Older People', in Silverman and Berzoff (2004).

Thompson, N. and Thompson, S. (2005) *Community Care*, Lyme Regis, Russell House Publishing.

Thompson, N. and Thompson, S. (2016) *The Social Work Companion*, 2nd edn, London, Palgrave Macmillan.

Thompson, S. (2002a) *From Where I'm Sitting*, Lyme Regis, Russell House Publishing.

Thompson, S. (2002b) 'Old Age', in Thompson (2002b).

Thompson, S. (2005) *Age Discrimination*, Lyme Regis, Russell House Publishing.

Thompson, S. (2009) 'Reciprocity in Crisis Situations', *Illness, Crisis & Loss* 17(1).

Thompson, S. and Thompson, N. (2008) *The Critically Reflective Practitioner*, Basingstoke, Palgrave Macmillan.

Thornicroft, G. (2006) *Shunned: Discrimination Against People with Mental Illness*, Oxford, Oxford University Press.

Ticktin, S. (1989) 'Obituary: R. D. Laing', *Asylum*, 4 (1).

Timonen, V. (2008) *Ageing Societies: A Comparative Introduction*, Maidenhead, Open University Press.

Todorov, T. (2009) 'Race and Racism', in Back and Solomos (2009).

Townsend, P. (2007) 'Using Human Rights to Defeat Ageism: Dealing with Policy-induced "Structured Dependency"', in Bernard and Scharf (2007).

UPIAS (1976) *Fundamental Principles of Disability*, London, Union of the Physically Impaired Against Segregation.

Valencia, R. R. (1997) *The Evolution of Deficit Thinking: Educational Thought and Practice*, London, Routledge.

REFERENCES

—. (2008) 'Islamic Feminism in India: Indian Muslim Women Activists and
Reform of Muslim Personal Law', *Modern Asian Studies* 42(2/3).

—, C., Scambler, S. and Bond, J. (2009) *The Social World of Older People:
Understanding Loneliness and Social Isolation in Later Life*, Maidenhead, Open
University Press.

Walker, A. (2009) 'Why Is Ageing So Unequal?', in Cann and Dean (2009).

Webb, S. (1989) 'Old Lesbians: Out and Proud', *Social Work Today*, 4 April.

Weber, M. (1930) *The Protestant Ethic and the Spirit of Capitalism*, London, George
Allen & Unwin.

Weber, M. (1947) *The Theory of Social and Economic Organization*, New York, Free
Press.

Weeks, J. (1986) *Sexuality*, London, Tavistock.

White, J. (2008) 'Family Therapy', in Davies (2008).

White, V. (2006) *The State of Feminist Social Work*, London, Routledge.

Wilkinson, R. G. (2005) *The Impact of Inequality: How to Make Sick Societies Healthier*,
London, Routledge.

Wilkinson, R. G. and Pickett, K. (2009) *The Spirit Level: Why More Equal Societies
Almost Always Do Better*, London, Allen Lane.

Williams, C. and Johnson, M. R. D. (2010) *Race and Ethnicity in a Welfare Society*,
Maidenhead, Open University Press.

Williams, C., Soydan, H. and Johnson, M. R. D. (eds) (1998) *Social Work and
Minorities: European Perspectives*, London, Routledge.

Williams, F. (1989) *Social Policy: A Critical Introduction*, London, Polity.

Williams, J. E. (2000) 'Race and Class: Why All the Confusion?', in Lang (2000).

Wilson, F. M. (2003) *Organizational Behaviour and Gender*, 2nd edn, Aldershot,
Ashgate.

Wilson, G. (2000) *Understanding Old Age: Critical and Global Perspectives*, London,
Sage.

Wise, S. (2000) 'Heterosexism', in Davies (2000).

Witcher, S. (2015) *Inclusive Equality: A Vision for Social Justice*, Bristol, The Policy
Press.

Wolfensberger, W. (1972) *The Principle of Normalization in Human Services*, Toronto,
National Institute on Mental Retardation.

Woodward, K. (ed.) (1997) *Identity and Difference*, London, Sage.

World Health Organization (1980) *International Classification of Impairments,
Disabilities and Handicaps: A Manual Relating to the Consequences of Disease*,
Geneva, World Health Organization.

Zartler, U. (2002) 'Poverty Risks and the Fight against Poverty', in Gruber and
Stefanov (2002).

INDEX